Pregnancy Diet Cookbook

A Complete Pregnancy Diet Cookbook for First Time Moms

BY

Stephanie Sharp

License Notes

Copyright 2021 by Stephanie Sharp All rights reserved.

No part of this Book may be transmitted or reproduced into any format for any means without the proper permission of the Author. This includes electronic or mechanical methods, photocopying or printing.

Table of Contents

Introduction

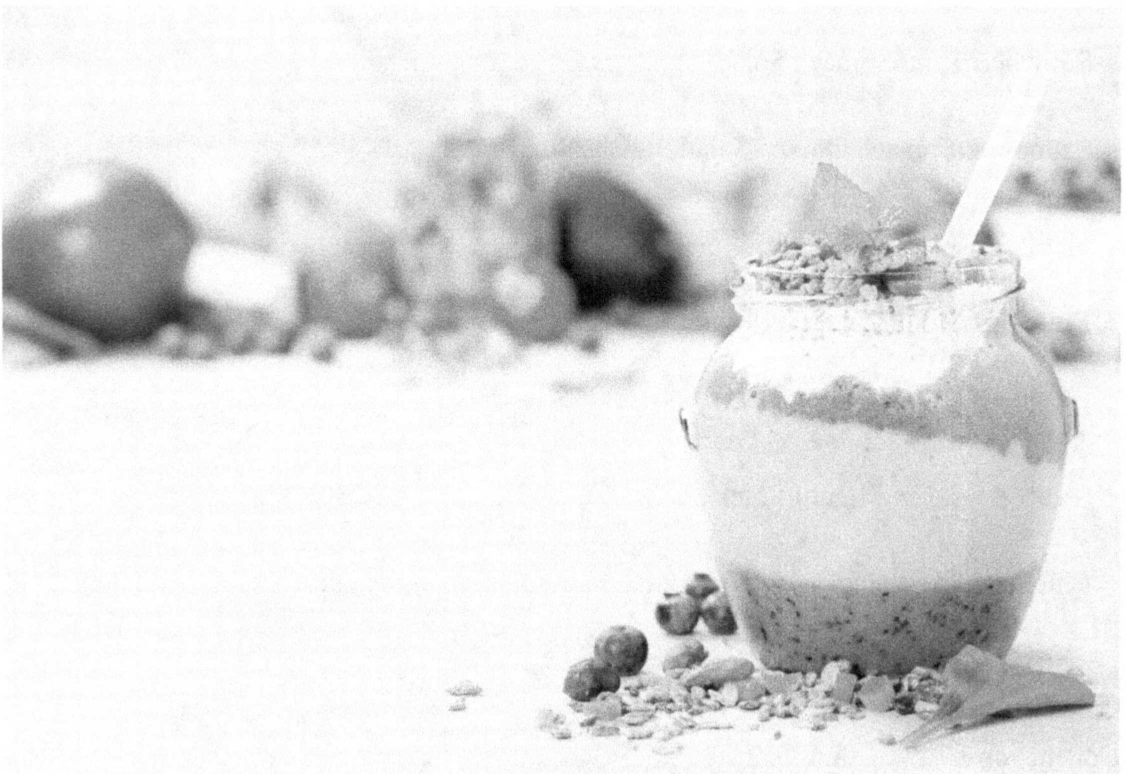

This e-book has plenty of tasty cooking ideas that you can try for the overall health of your baby who is living inside you.

It's strongly recommended that you don't pull anything heavy and spend a minimum of 1 hour in the sunlight throughout the pregnancy period. In addition to this, you need to maintain healthy blood pressure and sugar level as well.

For the first trimester, you need to ensure that you include more liquid in your diet. For this trimester, you can go for smoothies and easy to eat foods. Avoid recipes with meat or chicken.

For the other two trimesters, you can go for smoothies and other recipes mentioned in this book.

You get plenty of options to choose from, such as Spinach Berries Smoothie, Blueberry Smoothie, Almond Fruit Smoothie, Blueberry Veggie Smoothie, Raspberry & Banana Smoothie, Banana Walnut Pancakes, Mixed Sprouts Poha, Delicious Burritos, Spinach lamb wraps, Ginger Hoisin Chicken, Strawberry Spinach Salad, Banana Bread, Chicken and Broccoli, and so on.

Drinks/Smoothies

Superfruit Smoothie

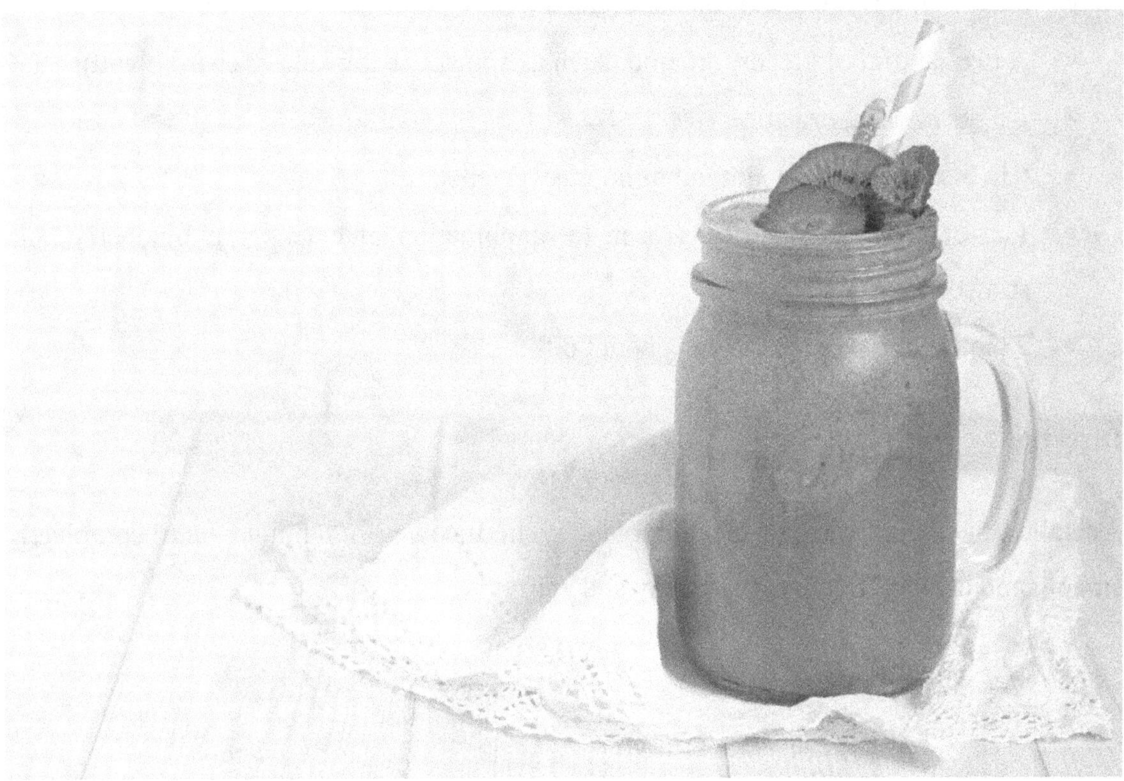

Prep Time: 5 minutes

Cooking Time: 5 minutes

Servings: 1 person

This gorgeous smoothie tastes great and is packed with all of the essential nutrients that you and your baby need. You can skip using flaxseeds and can add coconut milk than adding almond milk.

Ingredients

- 2 tablespoons flax hemp blend, organic
- A big handful of greens, organic (such as spinach, baby kale & chard blend)
- 1 large banana, organic
- 6 to 8 ounces vanilla almond milk, unsweetened
- 1 ½ cups organic berries, frozen (a combination of blackberry, blueberry, and strawberry)
- 2 tablespoon organic virgin coconut oil

Directions

Add all of the ingredients in a blender, blend on high power for a minute, until completely smooth and creamy. Serve immediately and enjoy.

Nutritional Value: kcal: 580, Fat: 34.2 g, Fiber: 12 g, Protein: 14 g

Spinach Berries Smoothie

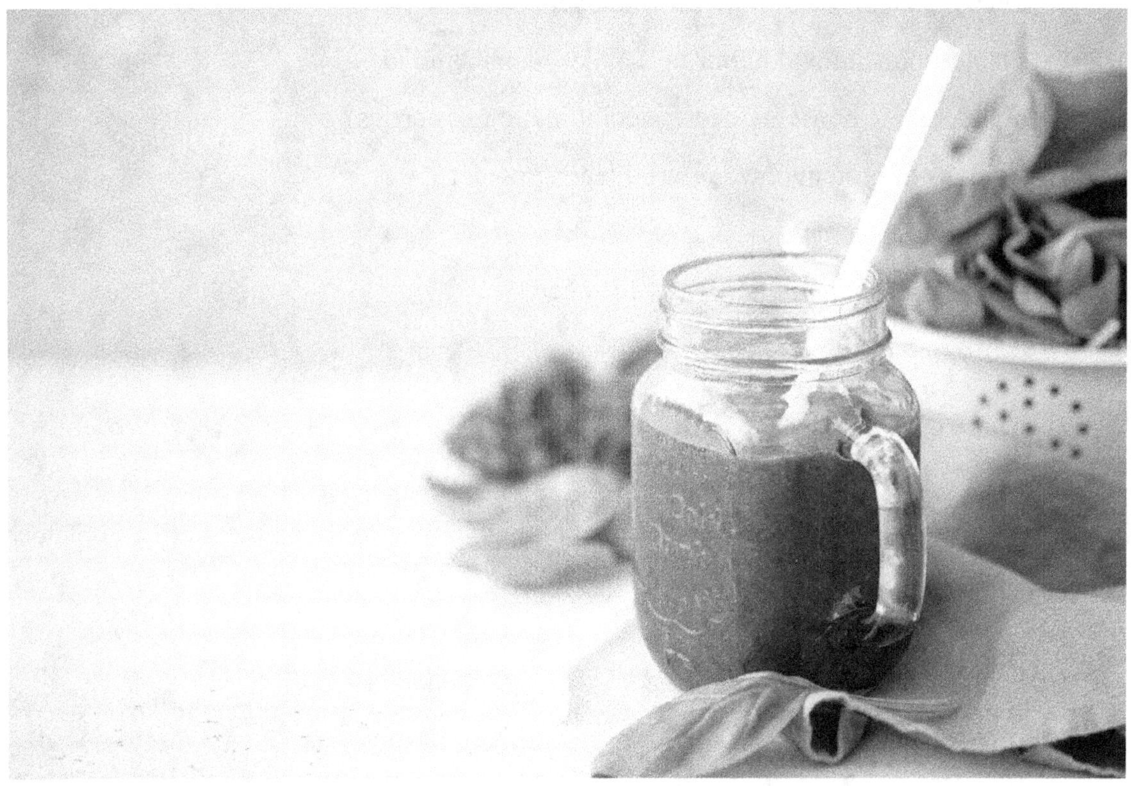

Prep Time: 5 minutes

Cooking Time: 5 minutes

Servings: 1 person

This drink would help you getting some greens when it's really hard to eat them during the first trimester. You can skip using banana, if desired.

Ingredients

- 2 cups mixed greens or organic spinach, fresh
- 1 tablespoon almond butter or 2 tablespoons almonds
- 1 cup organic berries, frozen (a combination of berries)
- 2 scoops of protein powder or collagen powder
- 1 tablespoon honey
- 1 cup vanilla almond milk, unsweetened
- ½ frozen banana

Directions

Add all of the ingredients in a blender, blend on high power for a minute, until completely smooth and creamy. Serve immediately and enjoy.

Nutritional Value: kcal: 420, Fat: 16 g, Fiber: 9 g, Protein: 19 g

Super-healthy Pregnancy Smoothie

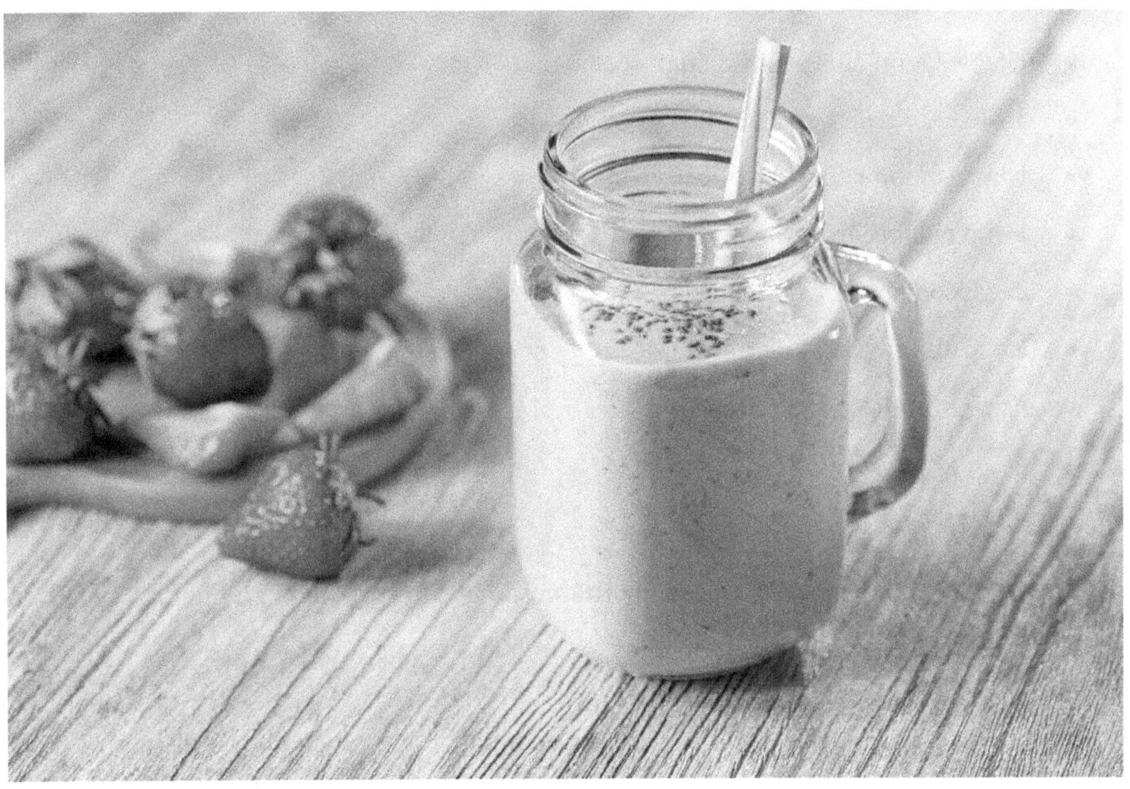

Prep Time: 5 minutes

Cooking Time: 5 minutes

Servings: 1 person

This smoothie is good for breastfeeding moms too. Spinach is optional. If you don't want to use It, then you can skip using it. Feel free to top your smoothie with grated almond.

Ingredients

- 1 cup raspberries, frozen
- 1 tablespoon chia seeds or flax seeds
- 3 Medjool dates, soft & pitted
- 1 tablespoon hemp seeds
- 1 cup mango, frozen
- 2 teaspoons DHA Oil, Udo's Choice
- 1 cup almond milk or water
- A handful of spinach, fresh

Directions

Add all of the ingredients (starting with 1 tablespoon of DHA oil) in a blender, blend on high power for a minute, until completely smooth and creamy.

Add the leftover DHA oil and blend again for a couple of more seconds. Serve immediately and enjoy.

Nutritional Value: kcal: 560, Fat: 20 g, Fiber: 19 g, Protein: 9 g

Blueberry Smoothie

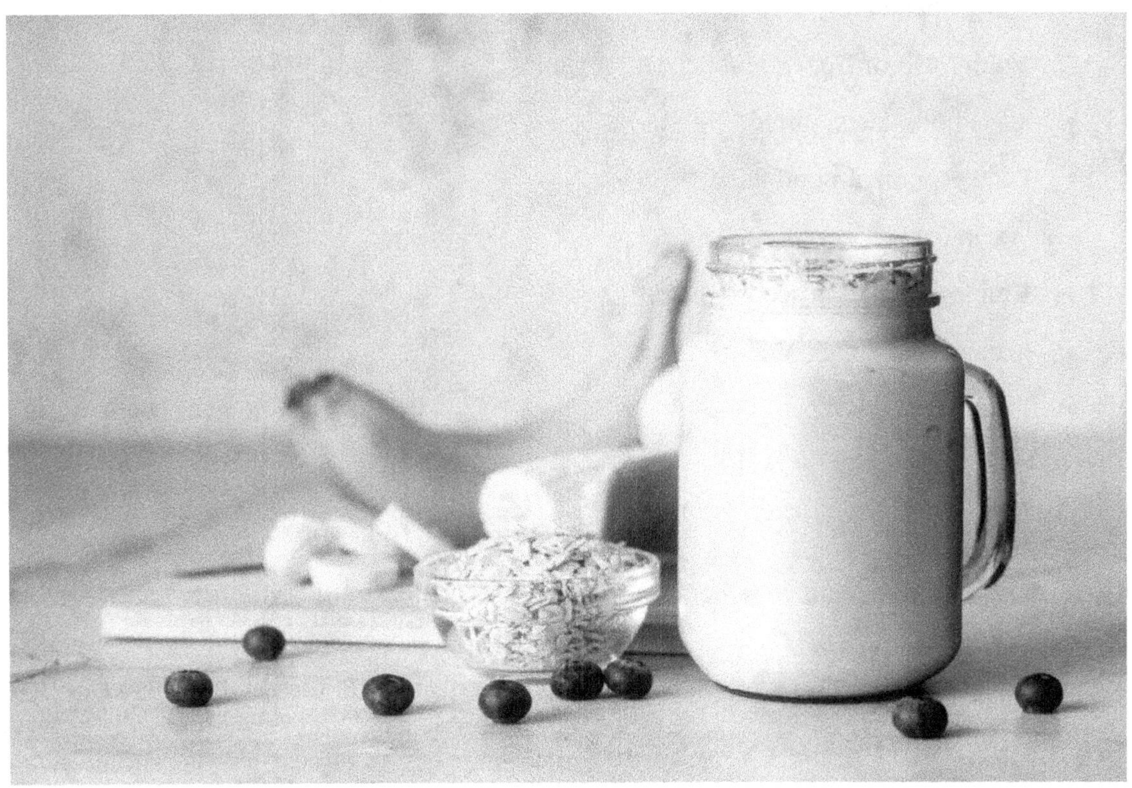

Prep Time: 1 minute

Cooking Time: 2 minutes

Servings: 2 persons

You can sub the Greek Yogurt with Vanilla Greek Yogurt.

Feel free to top your glass of smoothie with any of your favorites.

Ingredients

- 1 large banana
- 1 cup fresh or frozen blueberries, organic
- 3 Medjool dates, pitted
- 1 tablespoon almond butter
- ½ cup oat milk
- 1 tablespoon Chia seeds
- ½ cup plain Greek Yogurt
- 1 cup ice

Directions

Place all of the ingredients together in a blender, preferably in the order listed above.

Blend on high power until smooth and creamy. Evenly divide the mixture between two glasses, serve immediately & enjoy.

Nutritional Value: kcal: 333, Fat: 7.1 g, Fiber: 8.5 g, Protein: 10 g

Date Smoothie

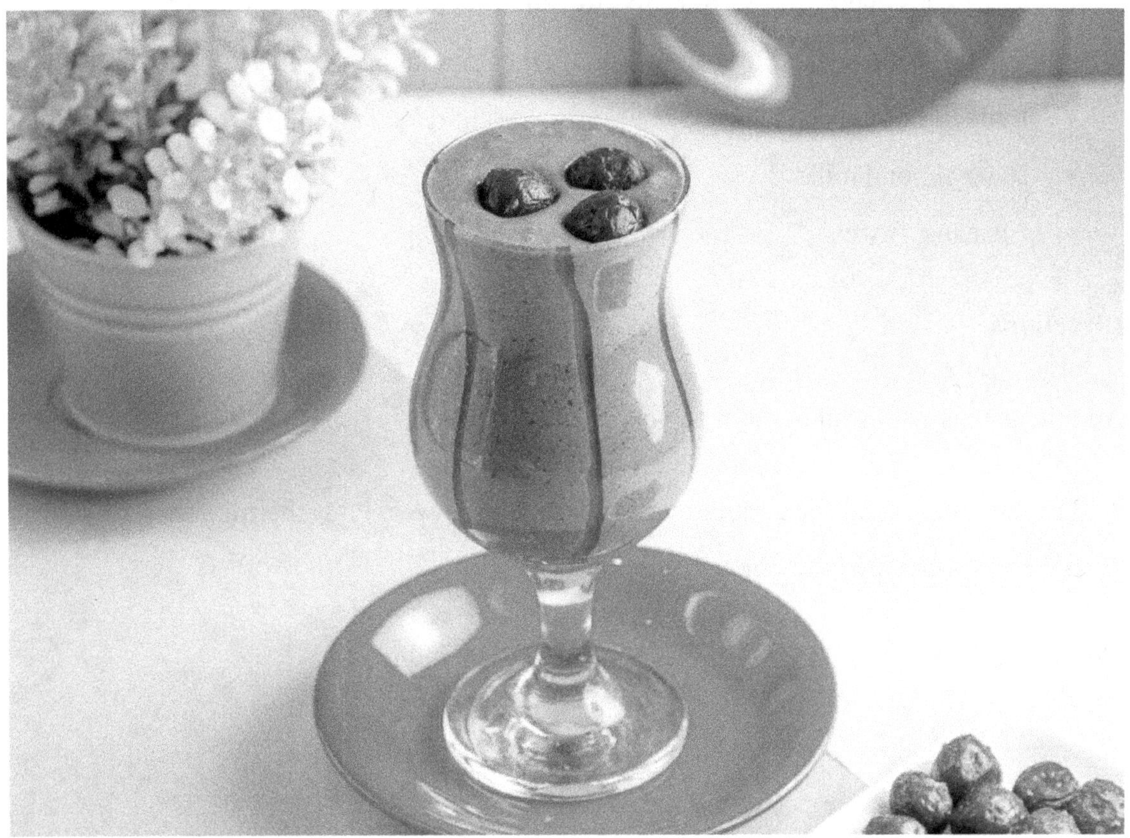

Prep Time: 5 minutes

Cooking Time: 5 minutes

Servings: 1 person

This smoothie is absolutely delicious and is really helpful during the final trimester. Feel free to sub the almond milk with any of your favorites and top your smoothie with fresh strawberries.

\

Ingredients

- 1 to 2 cups cherry berry fruit mix, frozen
- 4-6 date fruit, soaked in water for half an hour and then drain
- 1 cup of baby greens, mixed
- 16 oz almond milk
- 1 banana, frozen

Directions

Add the greens with fruit & dates to your blender.

Add in the milk, blend for a minute or two, on high power. Pour the mixture into a large glass, serve immediately & enjoy.

Nutritional Value: kcal: 650, Fat: 6 g, Fiber: 20 g, Protein: 12 g

Strawberry Banana Smoothie

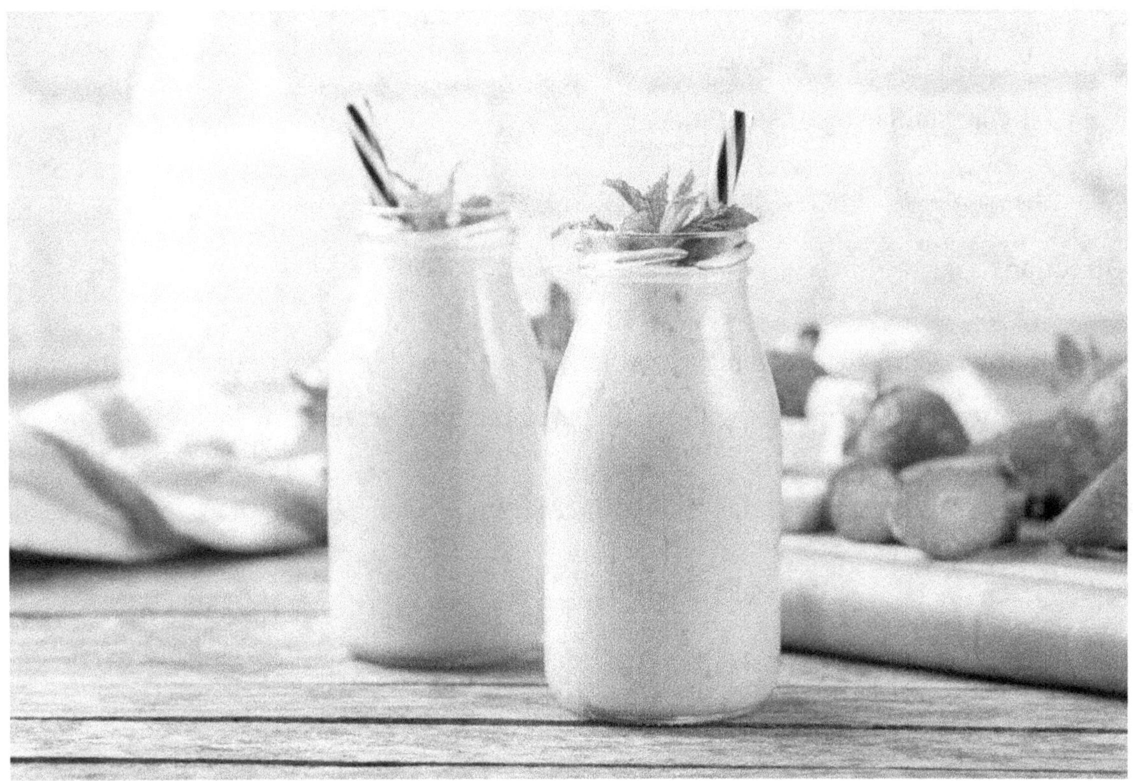

Prep Time: 2 minutes

Cooking Time: 2 minutes

Servings: 2 persons

Feel free to sub the skim milk with fresh orange juice. For added nutrition, just add a few spoonfuls of wheat germ mixed.

Ingredients

- 1 banana, sliced
- ½ cup strawberries, frozen
- 1 cup vanilla yogurt, nonfat
- ½ cup skim milk

Directions

Add all of the ingredients together in a blender, blend on high power until smooth, for a minute or two. Fill two glasses with the prepared mixture. Serve immediately & enjoy.

Nutritional Value: kcal: 176, Fat: 1.2 g, Fiber: 2.1 g, Protein: 8.1 g

Nutrient Packed Smoothie

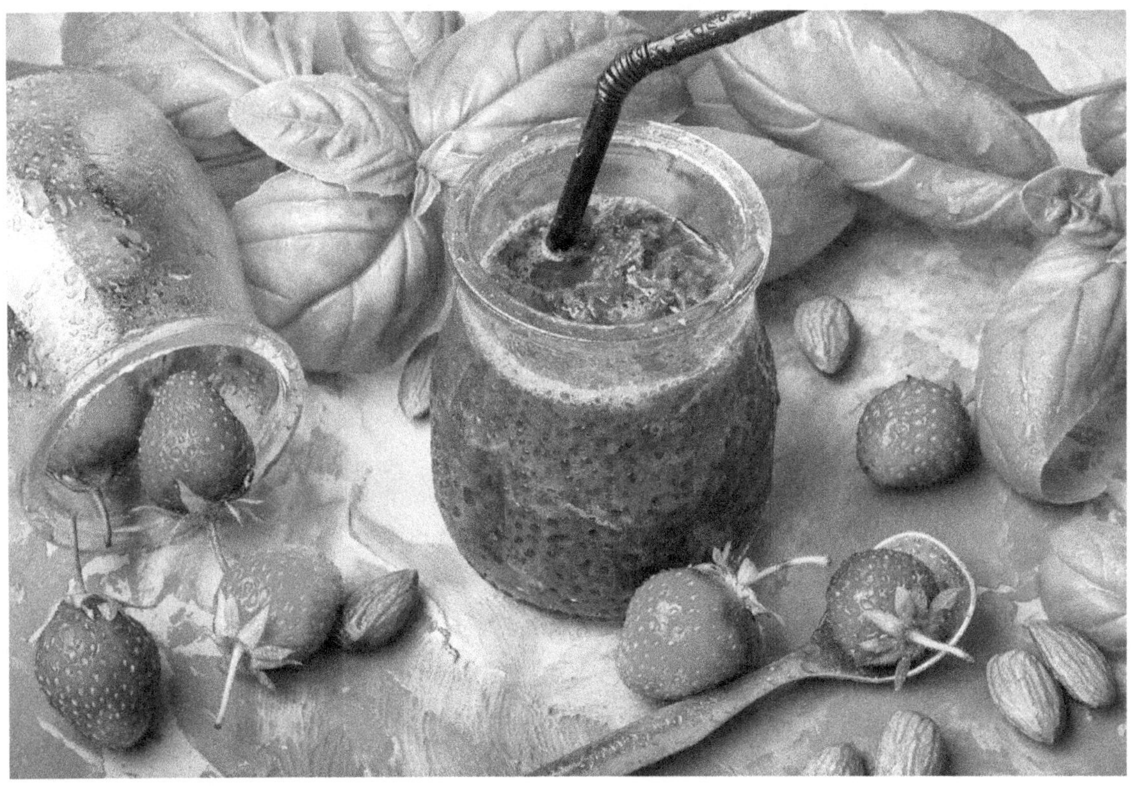

Prep Time: 2 minutes

Cooking Time: 5 minutes

Servings: 1 person

For instant nourishment, you must try this recipe. Feel free to top your smoothie with walnut and a fresh piece of strawberry.

Ingredients

- 30 oz coconut yogurt
- ½ cup vanilla almond milk, unsweetened
- 1 cup frozen strawberry halves, organic, sliced
- ¼ of a whole, ripe avocado
- 1 cup spinach, fresh
- 2 tablespoons chia seeds, soaked for half an hour
- 1 medium-sized banana, frozen & sliced

Directions

Add all of the ingredients to a Vitamix, process on high power until completely smooth & frothy. Serve immediately & enjoy.

Nutritional Value: kcal: 520, Fat: 14 g, Fiber: 16 g, Protein: 13 g

Almond Fruit Smoothie

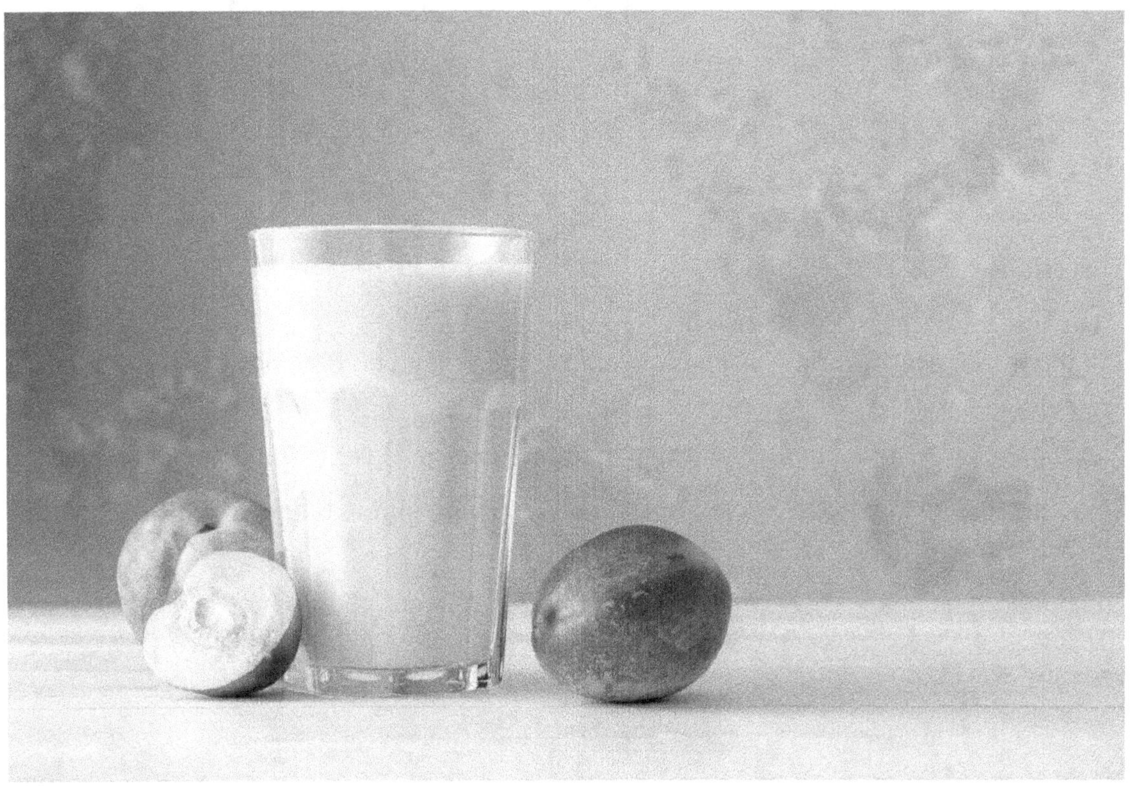

Prep Time: 5 minutes

Cooking Time: 5 minutes

Servings: 2 persons

Absolutely delicious and healthy! Feel free to top your drink with chocolate shavings, or mango slices, and even with a few blackberries.

Ingredients

- 2 tablespoons toasted slivered almonds
- 1 large banana, frozen, peeled & chopped
- 2 cups fresh orange juice
- 1 cup peaches, frozen

Directions

Put the frozen peaches and banana into your blender, blend on high power until smooth.

Next, pour in the orange juice and continue to blend until completely smooth. Pour the smoothie into a large glass. Serve immediately, top with almonds and enjoy.

Nutritional Value: kcal: 224, Fat: 3 g, Fiber: 3.2 g, Protein: 4.1 g

Green Pregnancy Smoothie

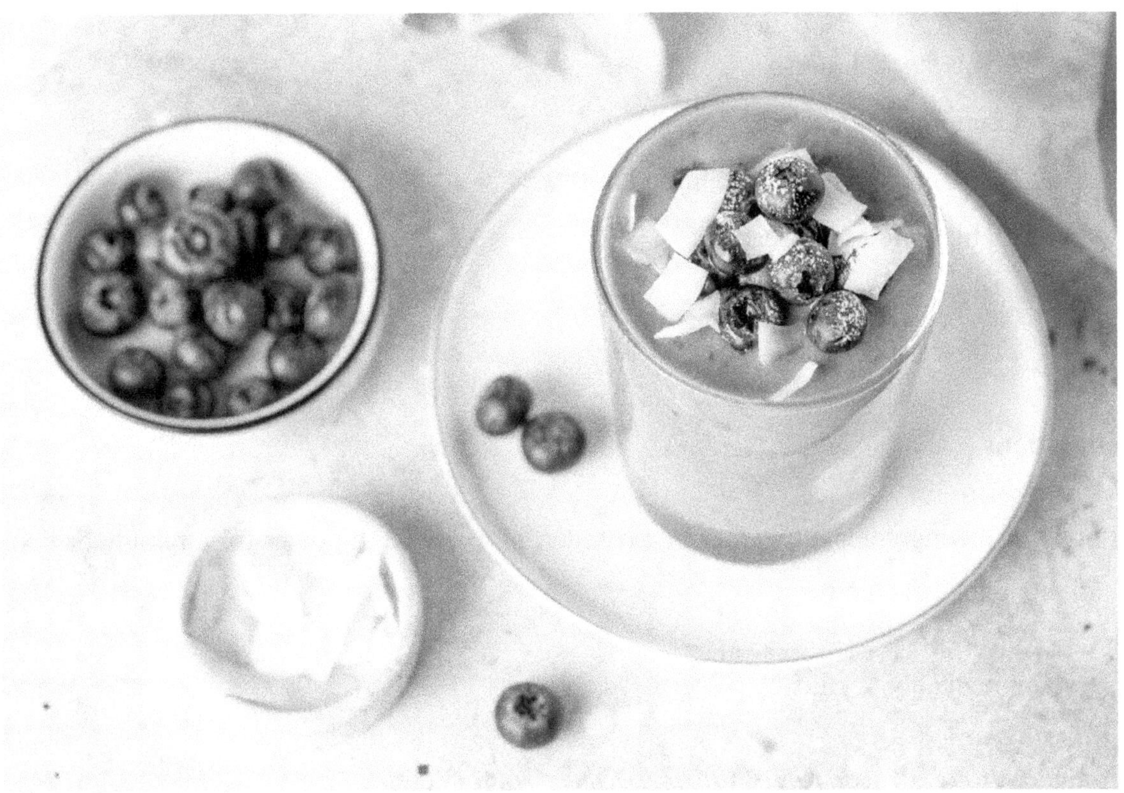

Prep Time: 5 minutes

Cooking Time: 5 minutes

Servings: 1 person

This smoothie is packed with all of the essential nutrients that your baby needs. Feel free to sweeten your drink a bit by adding a tablespoon or two of pure organic honey.

Ingredients

- 1 cup fresh raspberries
- 2 cups spinach, fresh
- 1 cup fresh blueberries
- 2 cups coconut water or almond milk
- 2 tablespoons chia seeds
- 1 large banana
- 1 cup fresh carrots

Directions

Put all of the ingredients together in a blender, puree on high power for a minute or two, until completely smooth.

Serve immediately & enjoy.

Nutritional Value: kcal: 541, Fat: 12 g, Fiber: 26 g, Protein: 11 g

Superfood-Powered Pregnancy Smoothie

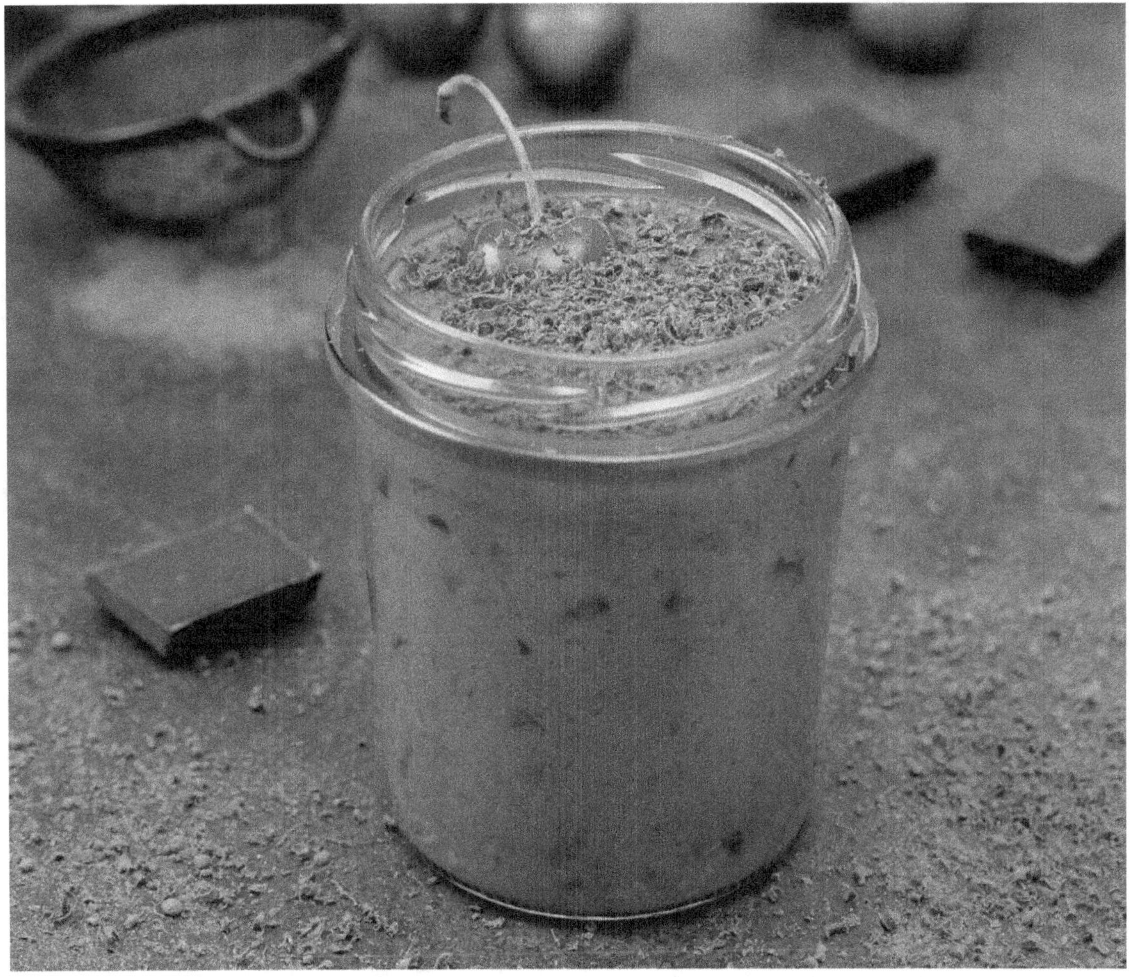

Prep Time: 2 minutes

Cooking Time: 5 minutes

Servings: 2 persons

A perfect drink for breakfast during pregnancy! Feel free to garnish your drink with your desired ingredients. Absolutely delicious and healthy!

Ingredients

- 1 tablespoon collagen peptides
- 1½ cups kefir
- 1 banana, frozen
- 1 teaspoon wheatgrass powder, freeze-dried
- ½ ripe avocado
- 1 tablespoon cacao nibs
- ½ cup blueberries
- 1 scoop vegan protein
- 5 strawberries, leaves removed
- 1 tablespoon goji powder
- 5 blackberries
- 1 tablespoon Jal Gua
- 5 raspberries
- 1 tablespoon baobab
- 1 teaspoon camu camu

Directions

Combine all of the ingredients together in a blender, blend on high speed for two to three minutes, until smooth.

Pour the prepared smoothie into a large glass.

Nutritional Value: kcal: 710, Fat: 22 g, Fiber: 16 g, Protein: 51 g

Chocolate Protein Smoothie

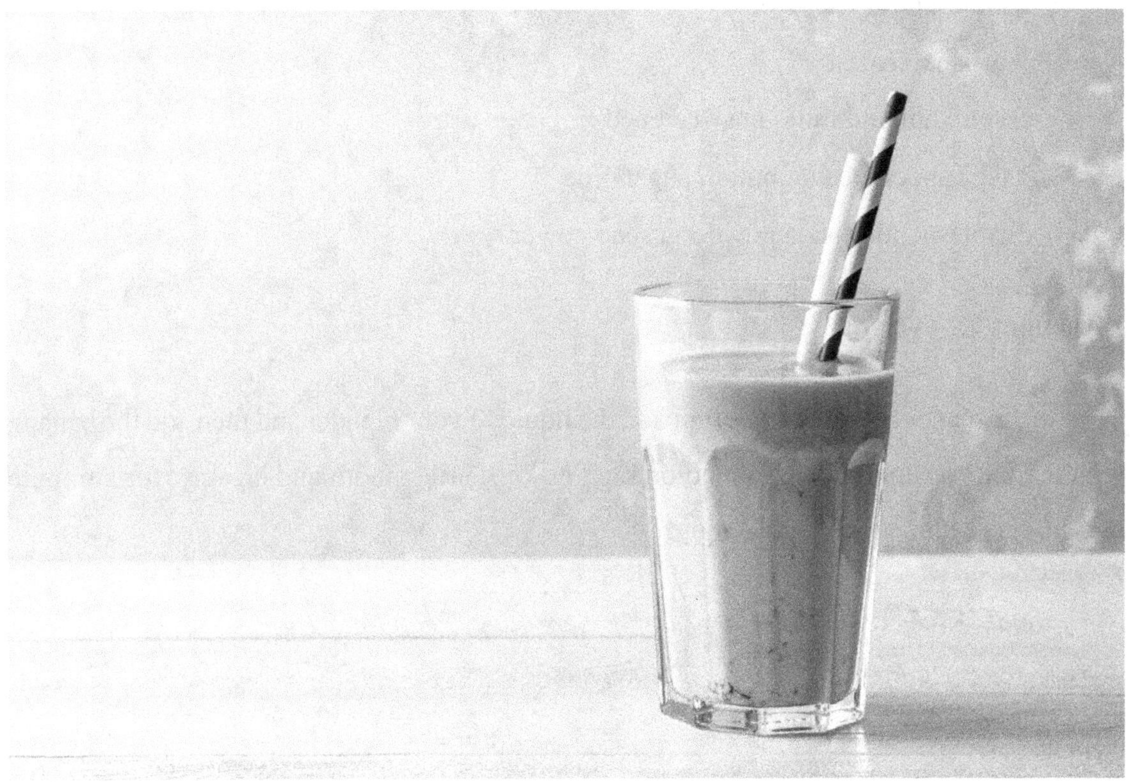

Prep Time: 5 minutes

Cooking Time: 5 minutes

Servings: 2 persons

One of the most delicious smoothie recipes that I have ever prepared! If desired, you can use gluten-free rolled oats for this smoothie.

Ingredients

- 2 tablespoons rolled oats
- 1 banana, frozen
- 500 ml almond milk, unsweetened
- 1 tablespoon peanut butter, sugar-free
- 2 tablespoons cocoa powder /cacao power

Directions

To stop the blades from sticking, first add the liquid to your blender and then add the banana with the leftover ingredients. Blend on high power until smooth and creamy, for a minute or two, serve immediately and enjoy.

Nutritional Value: kcal: 161, Fat: 7.0 g, Fiber: 4.0 g, Protein: 5.1 g

Anti Stretch-Mark Smoothie

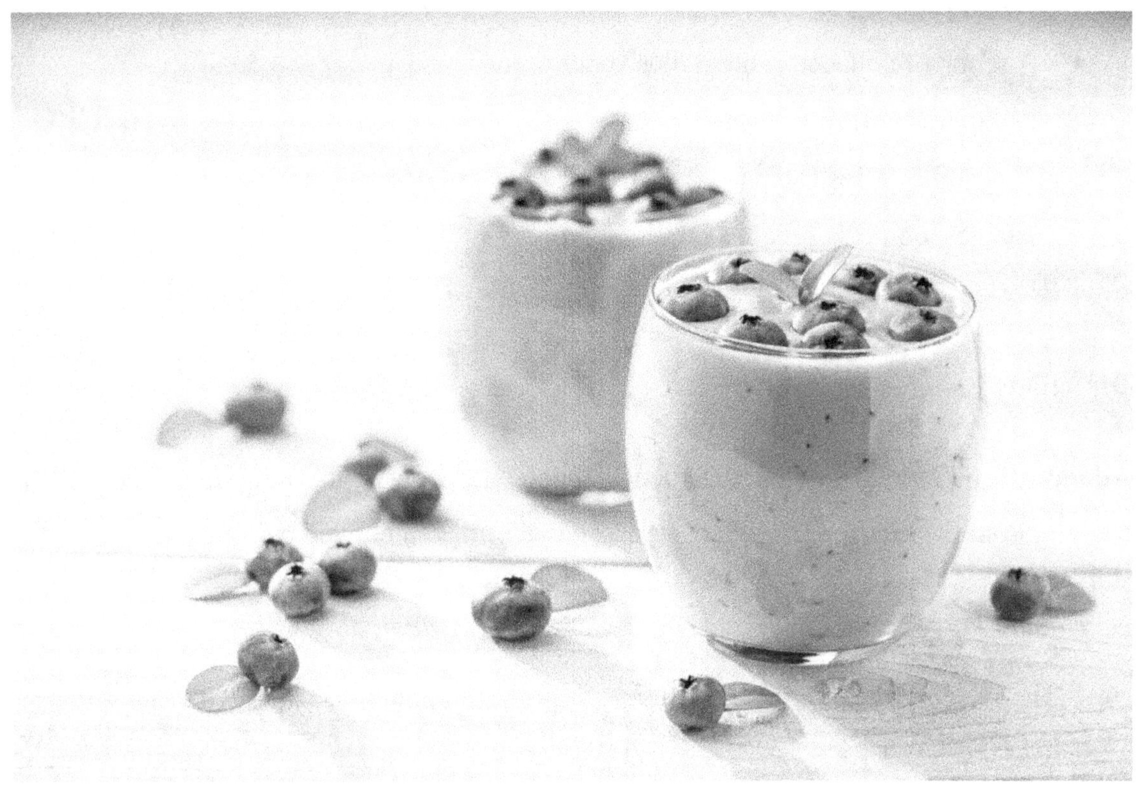

Prep Time: 5 minutes

Cooking Time: 5 minutes

Servings: 1 person

Just like the name, this smoothie would help you with the stretch marks that generally appear after the pregnancy. You can use raspberries or blueberries for this smoothie as well.

Ingredients

- ½ cup yogurt or goat kefir
- A scoop of collagen protein plus super greens
- ½ cup fresh blueberries
- A handful of fresh spinach
- 1 tablespoon chia seeds
- ½ ripe avocado

Directions

Add all of the ingredients together in a blender, blend on high power until smooth and creamy. Pour the mixture into a large glass, serve immediately and enjoy.

Nutritional Value: kcal: 785, Fat: 31 g, Fiber: 13 g, Protein: 80 g

Ginger Mint Strawberry Shortcake Prenatal Smoothie

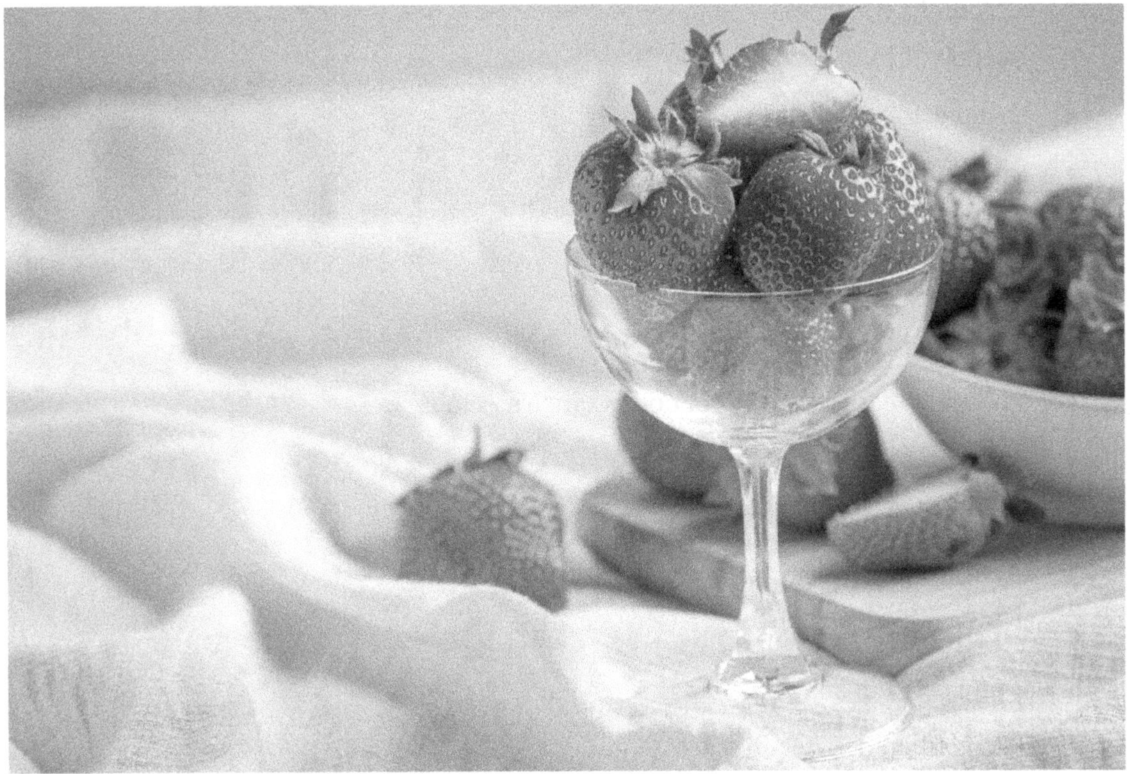

Prep Time: 5 minutes

Cooking Time: 5 minutes

Servings: 1 person

This smoothie is packed with everything that your body needs during the pregnancy period. You would fall in love with the color of this smoothie and would love the taste as well. Just before serving, garnish your drink with a few fresh mint leaves and enjoy.

Ingredients

- ½ of a ripe avocado
- 1 scoop of PureFood Iron
- ½ cup hemp seeds
- 1 Medjool Date, pitted
- ½ of a banana
- ¼ of a yam, baked
- ½ bunch of fresh mint leaves
- 1 heaping teaspoon of PureFood Women's A to Z
- ½ cup strawberries, frozen
- 1 tablespoon coconut oil
- ½ cup collard greens, steamed lightly
- 1 teaspoon Chia Seeds
- ¼ cup coconut shavings
- 2 cups filtered water
- ½ to 1" fresh ginger

Directions

Add all of the ingredients together (preferably in the order listed above) in a blender, blend on high power until smooth and creamy. Pour the mixture into a large glass, serve immediately and enjoy.

Nutritional Value: kcal: 551, Fat: 20 g, Fiber: 12 g, Protein: 42 g

Blueberry Veggie Smoothie

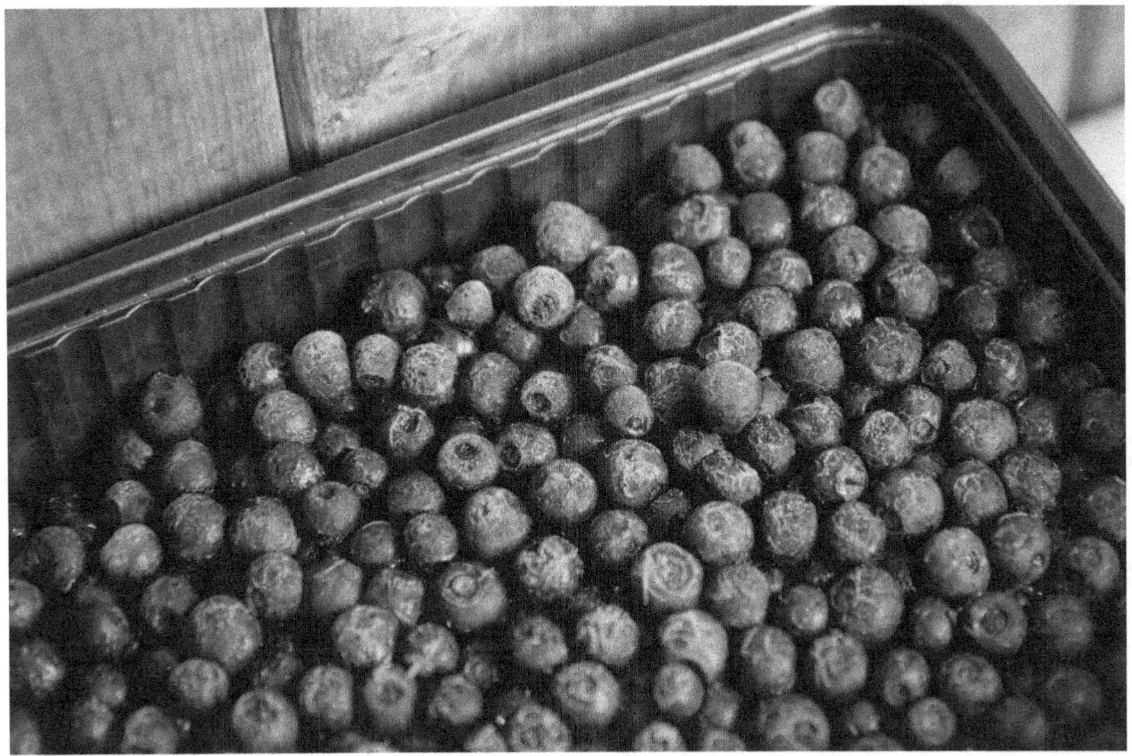

Prep Time: 5 minutes

Cooking Time: 5 minutes

Servings: 2 persons

You can use any of the non-dairy milk for this smoothie. Your body would get enough of fiber, healthy fats, and plant-based protein from this smoothie.

Ingredients

- 3 dates, pitted
- ¼ cup zucchini, frozen
- 2 handfuls of fresh spinach
- 1 cup blueberries, frozen
- 2 teaspoons bee pollen
- ¼ cup peas, frozen
- 2 tablespoons almond butter, raw
- 1 cup riced cauliflower, uncooked & frozen
- 3 tablespoons hemp seeds
- 1 ¼ cups almond milk, unsweetened
- ¼ avocado

Directions

Add the entire ingredients in a blender, blend until smooth & creamy, for a minute or two, on high power. Pour the prepared mixture into a large glass. Serve immediately, garnished with fresh blueberries & hemp seeds.

Nutritional Value: kcal: 413, Fat: 22 g, Fiber: 9 g, Protein: 19 g

Raw Banana Cacao Breakfast Smoothie

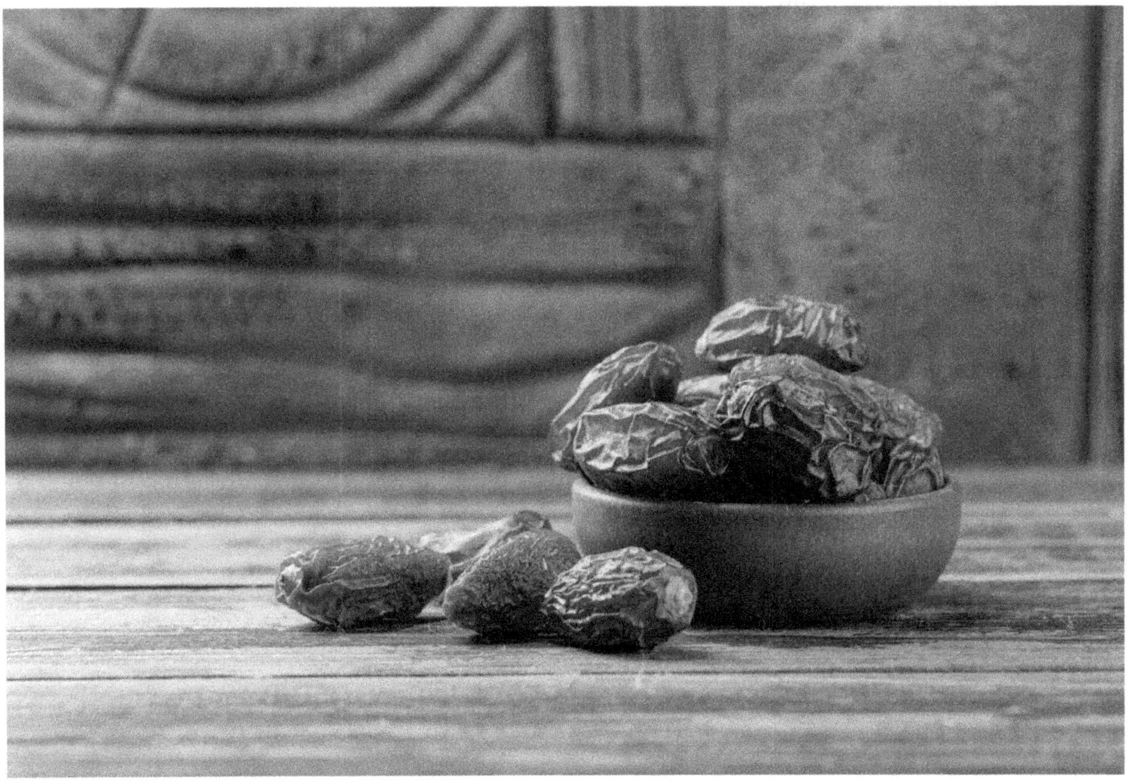

Prep Time: 5 minutes

Cooking Time: 5 minutes

Servings: 1 person

This recipe is so delicious that it would fill your mouth full of water. Packed with all of the essential nutrients, this breakfast smoothie recipe is a hit. You can top your drink with some of the cashew nut milk and can add more of date and some flaxseed powder.

Ingredients

- 2 Medjool dates, pitted
- 1 banana, frozen & sliced
- 2 tablespoons raw almond butter
- 1 tablespoon chia seeds
- 2 tablespoons raw cacao powder
- 1 cup almond milk, raw

Directions

Blend all of the ingredients together in a blender, on high power until smooth and creamy. Serve immediately and enjoy.

Nutritional Value: kcal: 344, Fat: 6 g, Fiber: 12 g, Protein: 6 g

Raspberry & Banana Smoothie

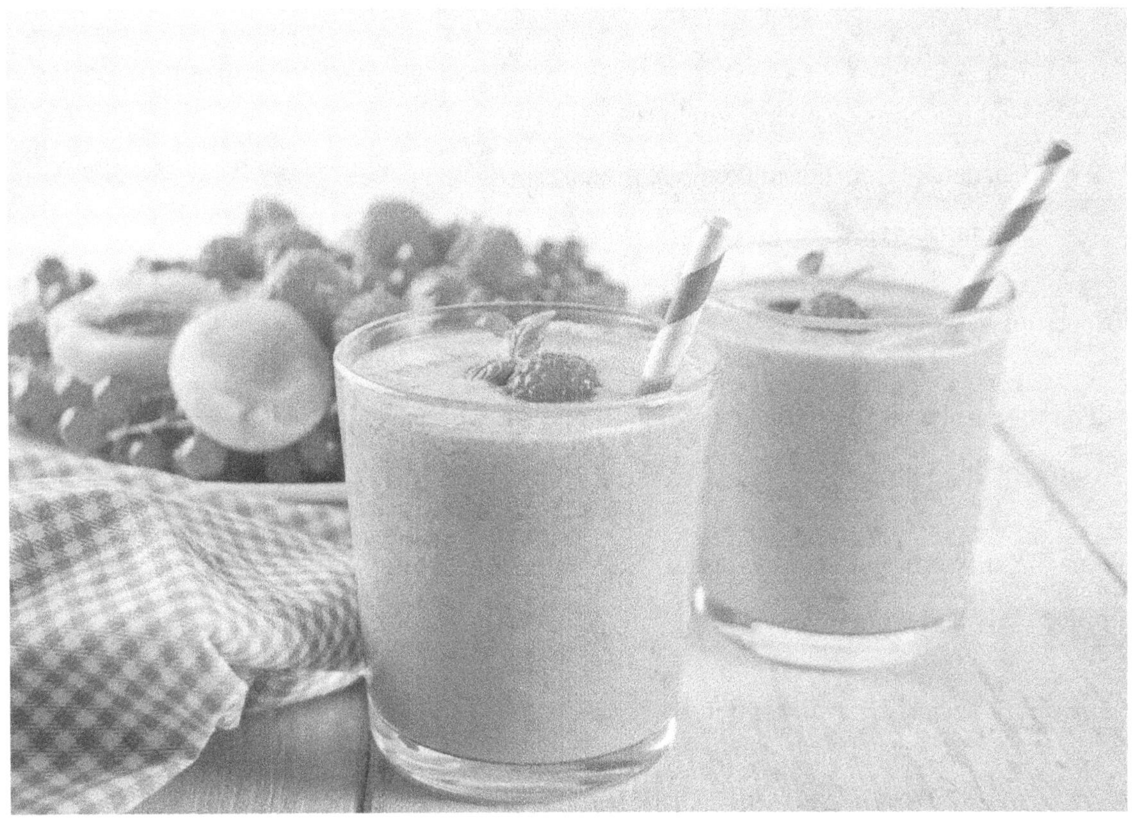

Prep Time: 5 minutes

Cooking Time: 5 minutes

Servings: 2 persons

You can surely love the fragrance of this recipe and would love the taste as well. Just before serving, you can top your glass with a few raspberries or banana slices.

Ingredients

- 50g strawberries, hulled & halved
- 1 teaspoon honey
- 3 tablespoons raspberry yoghurt
- 1 banana, large, cut into cubes, frozen
- 50g raspberries

Directions

Blend the raspberries with banana, yoghurt and strawberries in a blender until smooth and creamy, on high power.

Pour the mixture into large glasses, add some honey and give it a good stir. Serve immediately and enjoy.

Nutritional Value: kcal: 104, Fat: 0.6 g, Fiber: 3.7 g, Protein: 2.1 g

Breakfast Recipes

Banana Walnut Pancakes

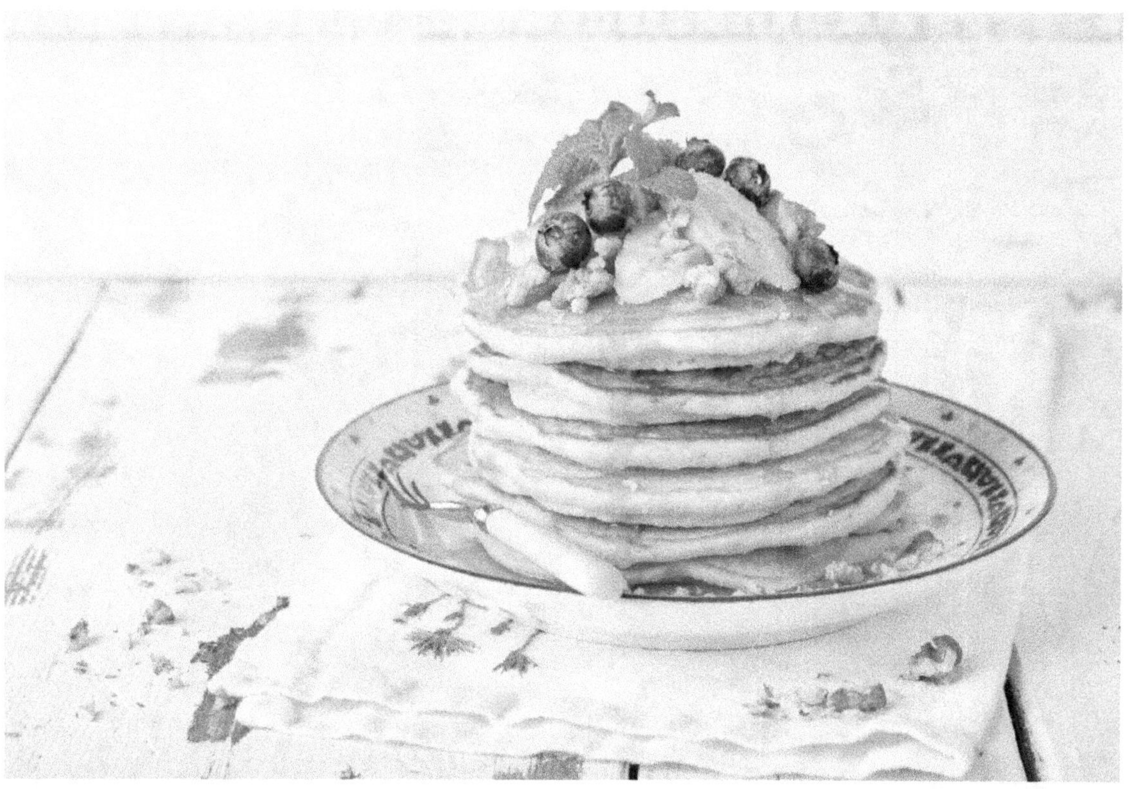

Prep Time: 10 minutes

Cooking Time: 20 minutes

Servings: 4 persons

You can sub the bananas with nectarines, ripe peaches (thinly sliced) or blueberries or even raspberries. Swap the walnuts with some pecans and use cacao nibs or carob chips than the chocolate chips.

Ingredients

- ½ cup whole wheat flour
- 1 cup all-purpose flour
- ½ teaspoon baking soda
- 3 tablespoons sugar
- 1 ½ cups buttermilk
- 2 organic eggs, large-sized
- ½ teaspoon vanilla extract
- 1 ripe banana, peeled & chopped
- ½ cup walnuts, chopped
- 1 teaspoon baking powder
- 3 tablespoons butter, melted & cooled slightly
- ¼ cup chocolate chips, semisweet
- 1 teaspoon salt

Directions

Preheat your griddle over medium heat in advance.

Next, whisk all of the dry ingredients together in a large-sized mixing bowl until mixed well.

Once done, whisk the buttermilk with vanilla, and eggs in a glass measuring cup. Slowly add & whisk butter into the prepared egg mixture.

Add the mixture of liquid ingredients into the mixture of dry ingredients & continue to mix using a wooden spoon or rubber scraper. Don't worry if there are still lumps in the batter.

For each pancake, pour approximately half a cup of the prepared batter on the griddle and then sprinkle with walnuts, bananas & the chocolate chips, lightly pressing the ingredients and ensure that they adhere. Cook until the edges start to turn dry & bottom turns golden brown, for a couple of minutes. Carefully flip & cook the other side for a couple of more minutes.

Serve the cooked pancakes with maple syrup and butter, if desired. Enjoy.

Nutritional Value: kcal: 519, Fat: 24 g, Fiber: 4.2 g, Protein: 12 g

Dal and Vegetable Idli

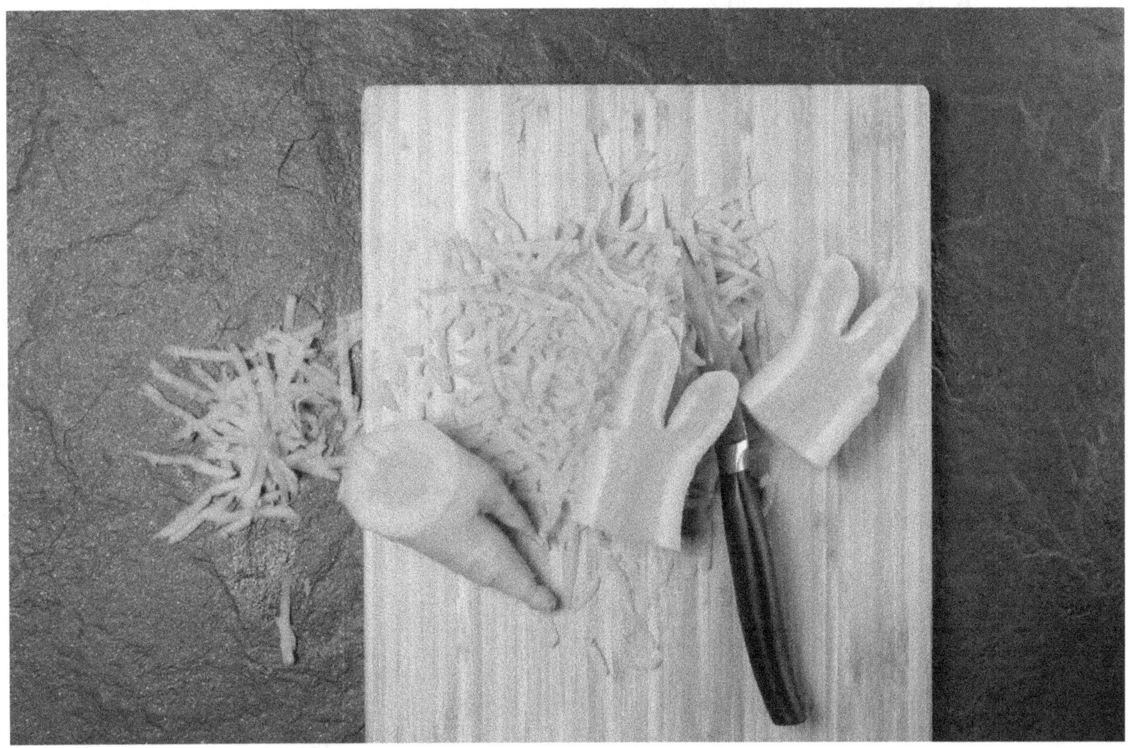

Prep Time: 10 minutes

Cooking Time: 30 minutes

Servings: 20 persons

If you are looking for an Indian-style pregnancy breakfast, then you must try this one. Absolutely delicious and perfect for pregnancy!

Ingredients

- ¼ cup green peas, boiled & mashed
- ½ cup arhar (toovar) dal
- ¼ cup coconut, grated
- 1 cup methi (fenugreek) leaves, chopped
- ½ cup split Bengal gram (chana dal)
- 2 cups coriander, chopped
- ¼ cup split yellow gram (yellow moong dal)
- 3 chopped green chilies
- ¼ cup carrot, grated
- 1 teaspoon oil
- ¼ cup onions, finely chopped
- Salt to taste

Directions

Wash & soak the dals for 3 hours (in enough water).

Drain & grind until you get smooth paste like consistency, feel free to add approximately ½ cup of water. Once done, immediately add in the coconut, green peas, coriander, fenugreek leaves, carrot, onion, green chilies and salt, mix the ingredients well

Add a bit of water, as needed and continue to knead until you get a thick batter like consistency.

Fill the idli moulds (preferably greased) with the prepared batter & steam until done, for 10 to 12 minutes.

Serve hot & enjoy.

Nutritional Value: kcal: 51, Fat: 1.1 g, Fiber: 1.9 g, Protein: 2.6 g

Delicious Spinach Dosa

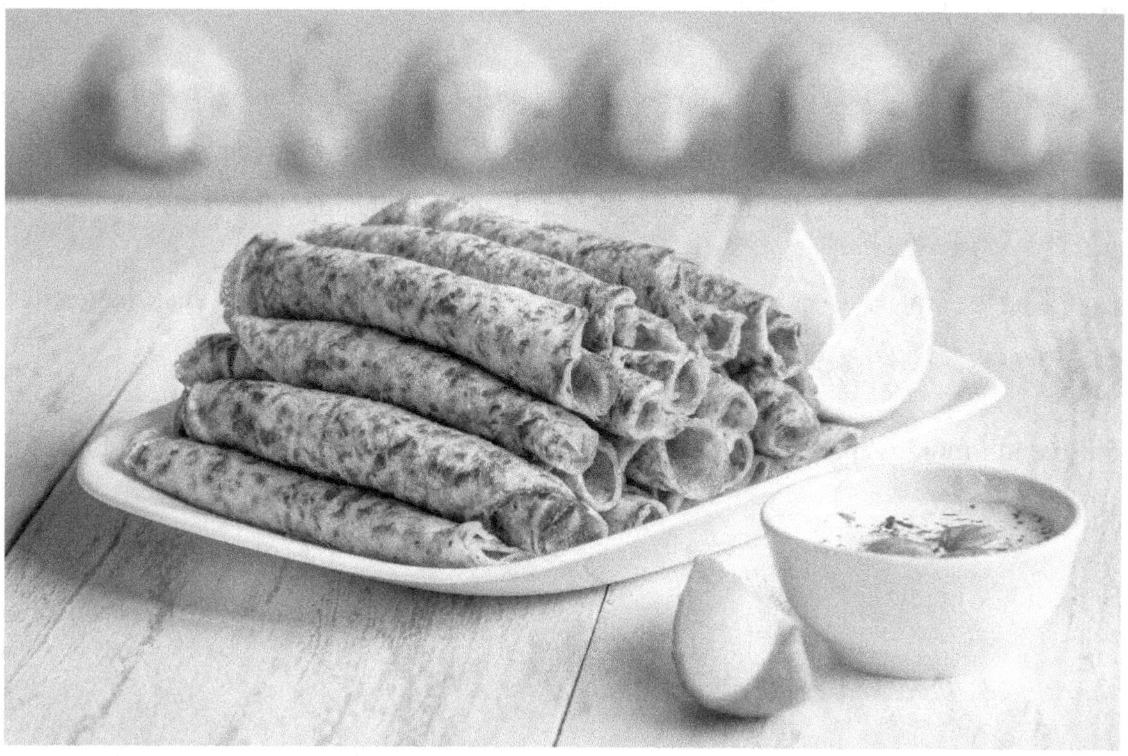

Prep Time: 20 minutes

Cooking Time: 25 minutes

Servings: 8 persons

Absolutely delicious and mouth-watering! This recipe will help you maintain a healthy haemoglobin level throughout the pregnancy.

Ingredients

- ½ cup spinach puree
- 1 cup whole wheat flour
- ¼ cup split black lentils
- 2 teaspoons oil
- ½ teaspoon fenugreek seeds
- Salt, as required, to taste

Directions

Soak the black lentils with fenugreek seeds in enough water for 2 hours. Once done, drain well

Add the soaked ingredients into a mixer and then add ½ cup of water, blend on high power until smooth.

Transfer the prepared mixture into a large, deep bowl and then add in the whole wheat flour followed by spinach puree, ½ cup of water and salt, mix well

Next, heat up a clean non-stick griddle over moderate heat.

Once done, pour a ladleful of the prepared batter on it and spread until you get a nice and thin circle.

Put approximately ¼ teaspoon of oil on it and spread, continue to cook until turns light brown

Serve immediately and enjoy.

Nutritional Value: kcal: 92, Fat: 1.6 g, Fiber: 3 g, Protein: 3.6 g

Beetroot Sesame Roti

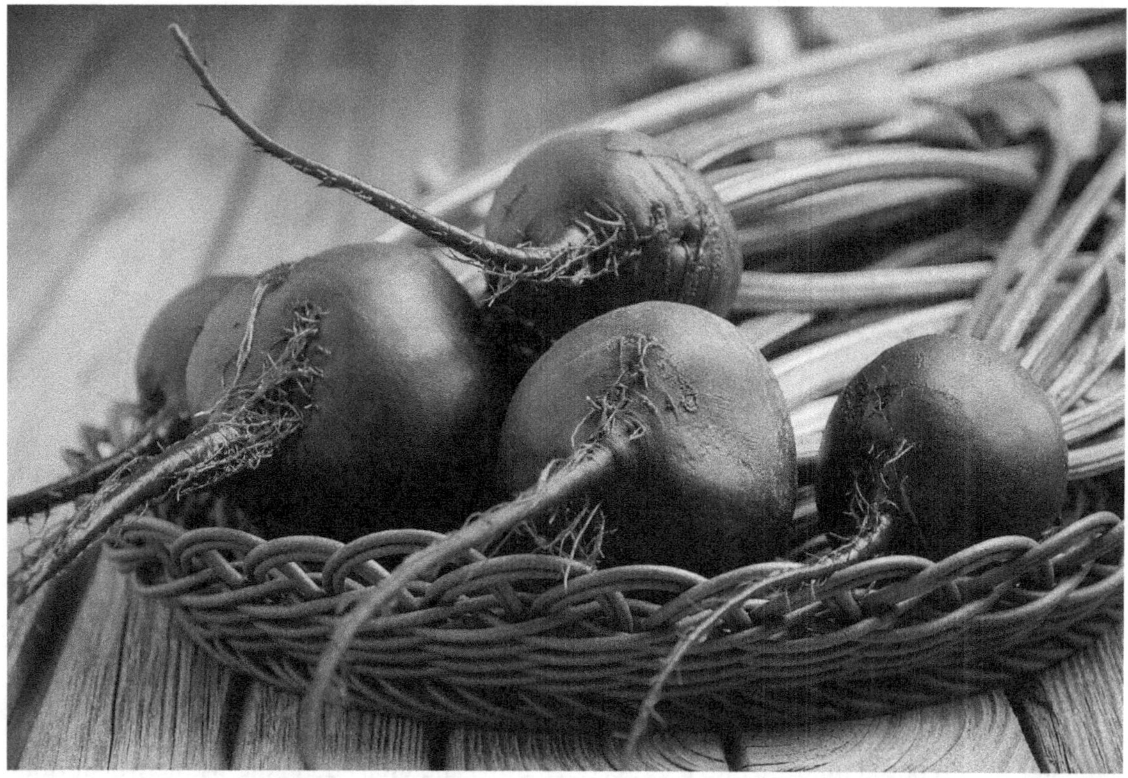

Prep Time: 10 minutes

Cooking Time: 20 minutes

Servings: 8 persons

This recipe is very famous in India. Just enjoy this recipe as a breakfast recipe. I normally serve mine with freshly prepared mint-chili chutney and some Cucumber Raita on the side.

Ingredients

- ½ cup whole wheat flour plus more for rolling
- 1 tablespoon sesame seeds
- ¼ cup beetroot, boiled, peeled & grated
- A pinch of asafoetida
- ¼ teaspoon turmeric powder
- 2 teaspoons oil
- ½ teaspoon coriander powder
- Salt to taste
- ½ teaspoon chili powder

Directions

Combine all of the ingredients together in a large-sized mixing bowl, knead until you get soft dough like consistency (feel free to add a bit of water, as required)

Evenly divide the prepared dough into eight portions and roll each portion out into 4" diameter (feel free to use a bit of wheat flour for rolling)

Next, over moderate heat in a large, non-stick griddle, cook each roti with approximately 1/4 teaspoon of oil until turn golden brown on both sides.

Set aside and let cool. Serve and enjoy.

Nutritional Value: kcal: 54, Fat: 3.1 g, Fiber: 1.1 g, Protein: 1.1 g

Mixed Sprouts Poha

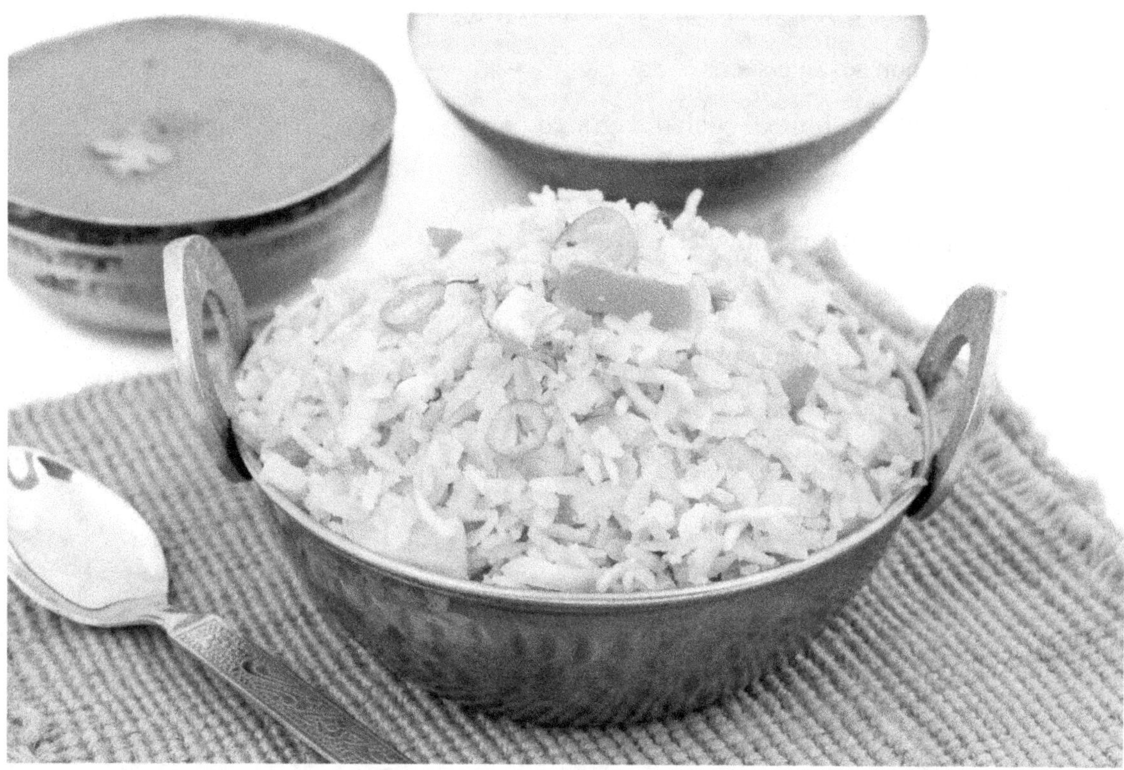

Prep Time: 10 minutes

Cooking Time: 10 minutes

Servings: 4 persons

This recipe has an amazing taste and quite easy to prepare. If you are looking for something light but yet tasty in the breakfast, then I recommend you to go for this one.

Ingredients

- 1 ½ cups poha (beaten rice)
- ½ cup onions, finely chopped
- 1 tablespoon lemon juice, fresh
- 1 ½ cups mixed sprouts, boiled
- ½ teaspoon mustard seeds
- 1 tablespoon green chilies, finely chopped
- ½ teaspoon turmeric powder
- 1 teaspoon peanut oil
- Salt, as required, to taste
- 1 tablespoon fresh coriander, finely chopped

Directions

Place the poha on a sieve and wash it lightly, drain and set aside for a couple of minutes.

Next, over moderate heat in a large, non-stick pan, heat up the oil until hot and then add the mustard seeds.

Cook until the seeds start to crackle. Once done, immediately add and sauté the onions and green chilies until the onion turn light brown in color, for a couple of minutes.

Add in the mixed sprouts, mix well and continue cooking for a minute or two more.

Add turmeric powder and salt, mix well and continue to cook for a minute.

Add approximately ¼ cup of water, mix the ingredients & cook for a minute or two more.

Add in the lemon juice, and poha, continue to cook for two more minutes, stirring frequently.

Serve hot, garnished with freshly chopped coriander and enjoy.

Nutritional Value: kcal: 156, Fat: 2 g, Fiber: 3.2 g, Protein: 5.2 g

Strawberry Oatmeal Bars

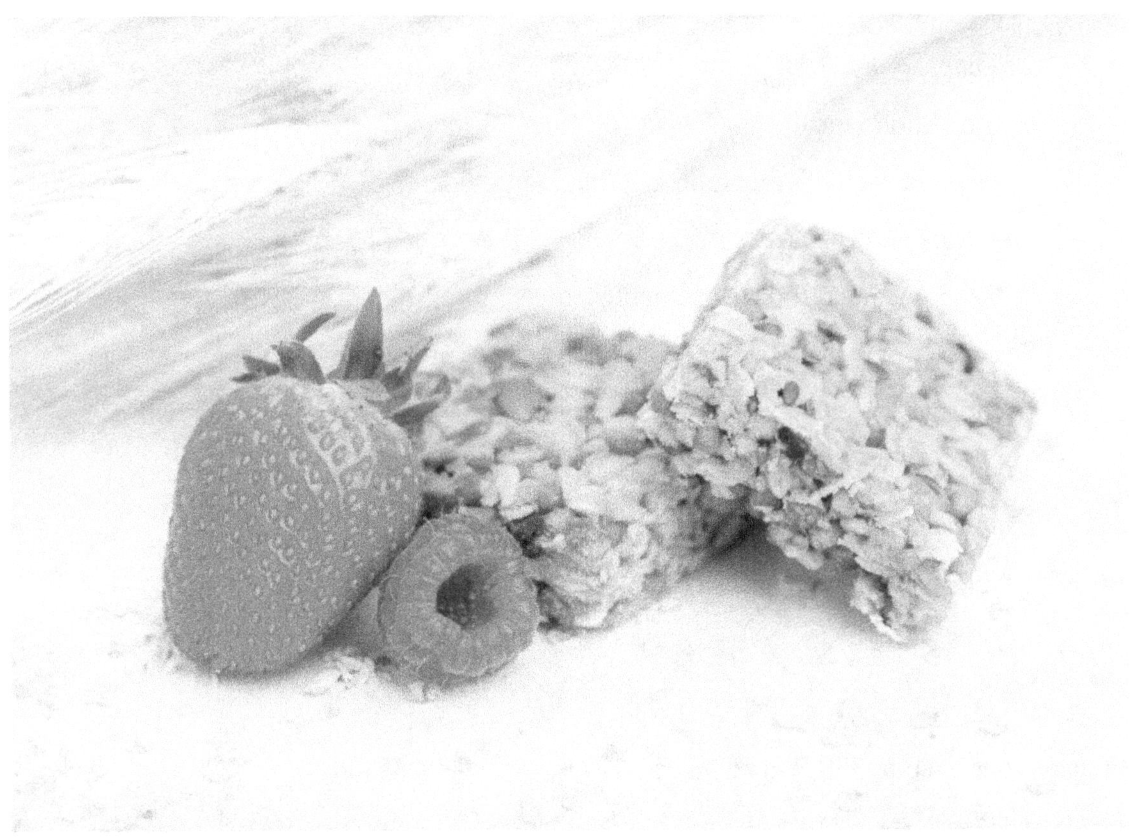

Prep Time: 30 minutes

Cooking Time: 50 minutes

Servings: 4 persons

This recipe is so delicious that you wouldn't be able to control yourself. You can sub the almond milk with oat milk, cashew milk, or any of your favorite non-dairy milk. You can even use freeze-dried bananas, fresh berries, walnuts, shredded coconut, chocolate chips, and almonds in this recipe.

Ingredients

- ¼ cup strawberries, freeze-dried
- 2 ½ cups oatmeal
- ½ cup almond meal
- 1 teaspoon each of cinnamon, and baking powder
- 3 tablespoons chia seeds
- 1 ½ cups Almond milk plus 2 tablespoons more
- 2 scoops of protein powder (only designed for pregnancy)
- ¼ cup agave nectar
- 1 banana, large-sized, mashed
- 2 tablespoons softened almond butter
- 1 tablespoon vanilla extract

Directions

Preheat your oven to 350 F in advance.

In the meantime, mash & combine the banana with almond butter, extract, agave and milk until mixed well. Add in the leftover ingredients (except the strawberries) & continue to combine the ingredients until mixed well.

Fold in the strawberries.

Pour the mixture into an 8" square pan (lightly greased with the coconut oil) & bake in the preheated oven for 30 to 35 minutes.

Nutritional Value: kcal: 430, Fat: 16 g, Fiber: 9 g, Protein: 21 g

Blueberry Oatmeal Muffins

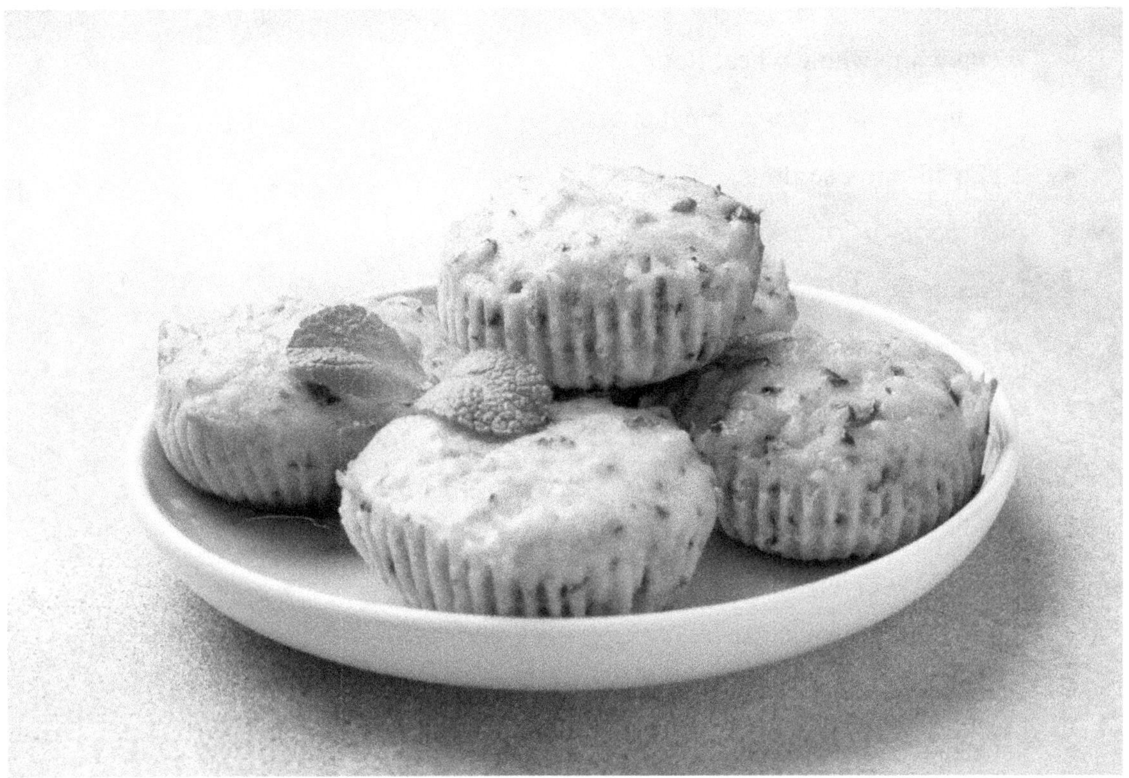

Prep Time: 10 minutes

Cooking Time: 40 minutes

Servings: 16 persons

Rather than using the wheat germ, you can use the oat bran. Feel free to use coconut palm sugar in this recipe. Just serve these delicious muffins with a glass full of almond milk and enjoy.

Ingredients

- ½ cup milk, low-fat
- ¾ cup white whole wheat flour
- 1 ½ cups fresh or frozen blueberries
- ¾ cup all-purpose flour
- 2 teaspoons baking soda
- 1 ½ cups quick-cooking oats
- ½ teaspoon baking powder
- ½ cup wheat germ
- 1 ½ teaspoons cinnamon
- 1/3 cup safflower oil
- 1 organic egg, large-sized
- ¾ cup light brown sugar
- 1 cup vanilla Greek yogurt, reduced-fat
- ½ teaspoon kosher salt

Directions

Line 2 muffin tins (12-cups each) with 16 paper muffin liners and then preheat your oven to 375 F in advance.

Next, combine oats with flours, sugar, wheat germ, baking powder, baking soda, cinnamon & salt in a large-sized mixing bowl until mixed well.

Combine the yogurt with egg, oil, and milk in a separate bowl.

Add the mixture of wet ingredients into the mixture of dry ingredients, give it a good stir until combined (ensure that you don't over-mix the ingredients). Gently stir blueberries into the prepared batter.

Next, fill each muffin cups approximately ¾ full with the prepared batter.

Bake in the preheated oven until a toothpick comes out clean and the muffins turn golden brown, for 17 to 20 minutes.

Let cool for 5 to 10 minutes in the pan and then carefully turn the muffins out onto a rack & let completely cool. Serve immediately and enjoy.

Nutritional Value: kcal: 170, Fat: 4 g, Fiber: 2.4 g, Protein: 4.6 g

Daliya Upma

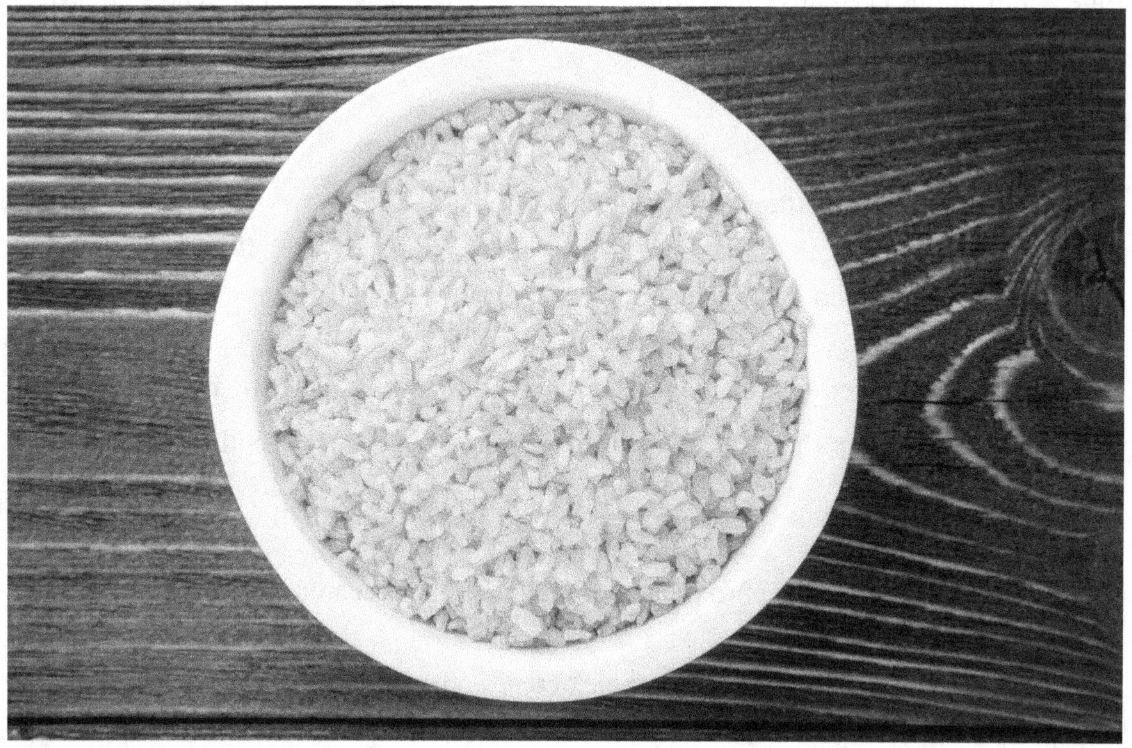

Prep Time: 10 minutes

Cooking Time: 20 minutes

Servings: 2 persons

My grandmother used to cook this recipe for me when I was expecting it for the first time. Serve hot with some tea or coffee on the side and enjoy.

Ingredients

- ¼ cup peas
- 1 ½ cups dalia (broken wheat), thoroughly washed under running water, drained well
- ½ teaspoon mustard seeds
- 1 green chili, medium-sized
- ½ medium onion, chopped
- 1 ½ teaspoons olive oil
- ½ teaspoon ginger, grated
- 2 ½ cups water
- ¼ cup carrot, diced

For Garnish:

- A handful of fresh coriander leaves, chopped

Directions

Over moderate heat in a pressure cooker, heat up the olive oil for a minute, until hot and then add the mustard seeds, cook until begin to splutter. Once done, immediately add in the onions, ginger and green chili, sauté until the onions turn slightly pink, for a minute or two.

After a couple of seconds, add in the green peas followed by broken wheat, carrots & salt, give the ingredients a good stir. Decrease the heat to low and sauté the ingredients for 3 to 4 minutes.

Add 2 ½ cups of water & pressure cook until you heat a whistle. Once done, turn the flame off & transfer the ingredients into a large-sized serving bowl. Serve hot, garnished with freshly chopped coriander leaves.

Nutritional Value: kcal: 447, Fat: 6.2 g, Fiber: 19 g, Protein: 22 g

Delicious Burritos

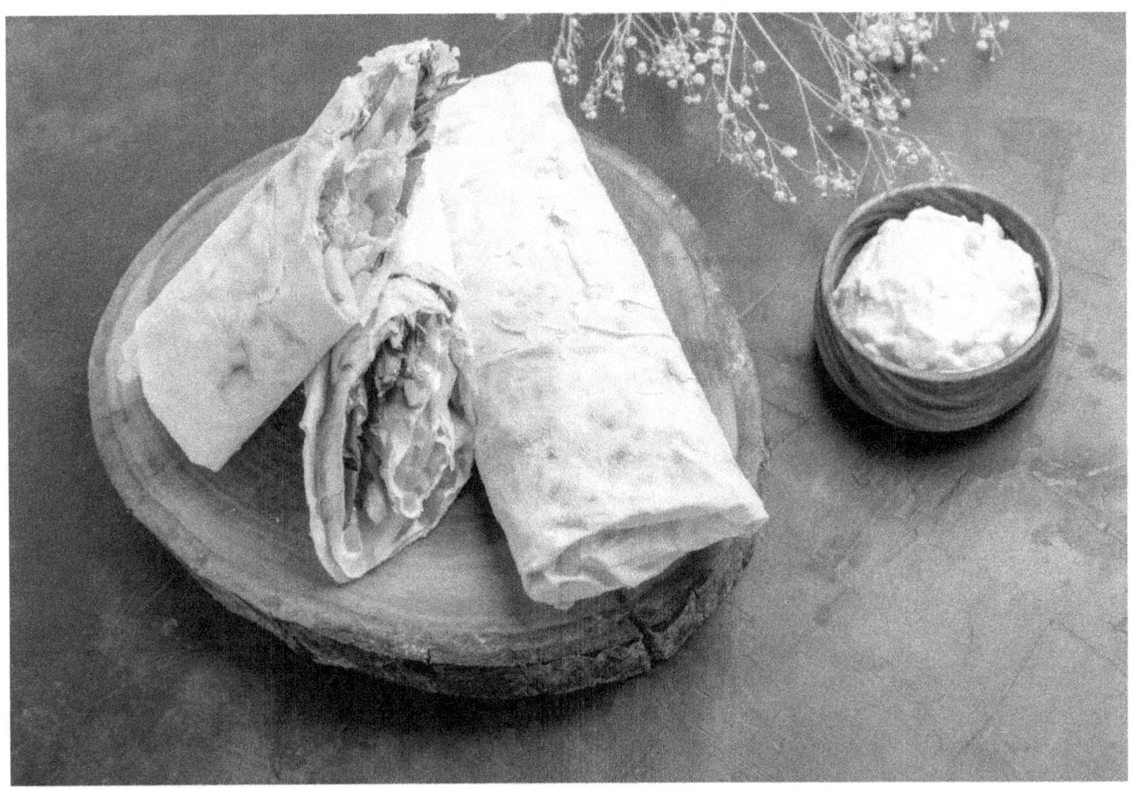

Prep Time: 10 minutes

Cooking Time: 10 minutes

Servings: 1 person

Absolutely delicious and healthy! For added nutrition, feel free to add a few slices of ripe avocado.

Ingredients

- ¼ cup tomato, chopped & deseeded
- 1 flour tortilla
- ¼ cup warmed refried beans
- 5 to 6 sliced black olives
- ¼ cup warmed seasoned taco meat
- 2 to 3 tablespoons sour cream
- ¼ cup shredded sharp cheddar cheese
- 1 to 2 green onion, sliced
- ¼ cup fresh lettuce, coarsely shredded or thinly sliced
- Taco sauce to taste

Directions

Warm the burrito skin and then place it on a microwave-safe serving plate.

Next, spread the beans down the middle of your burrito and then top with the cheese, taco meat, olives, tomato, onions and sour cream.

Cook in the microwave on high power for a minute, until the cheese starts to melt & bubble up.

Sprinkle with the lettuce & dash of the taco sauce, roll up & place on the plate, seam-side down. Serve and enjoy.

Nutritional Value: kcal: 270, Fat: 20 g, Fiber: 1.9 g, Protein: 6.4 g

Baobab Yogurt Breakfast

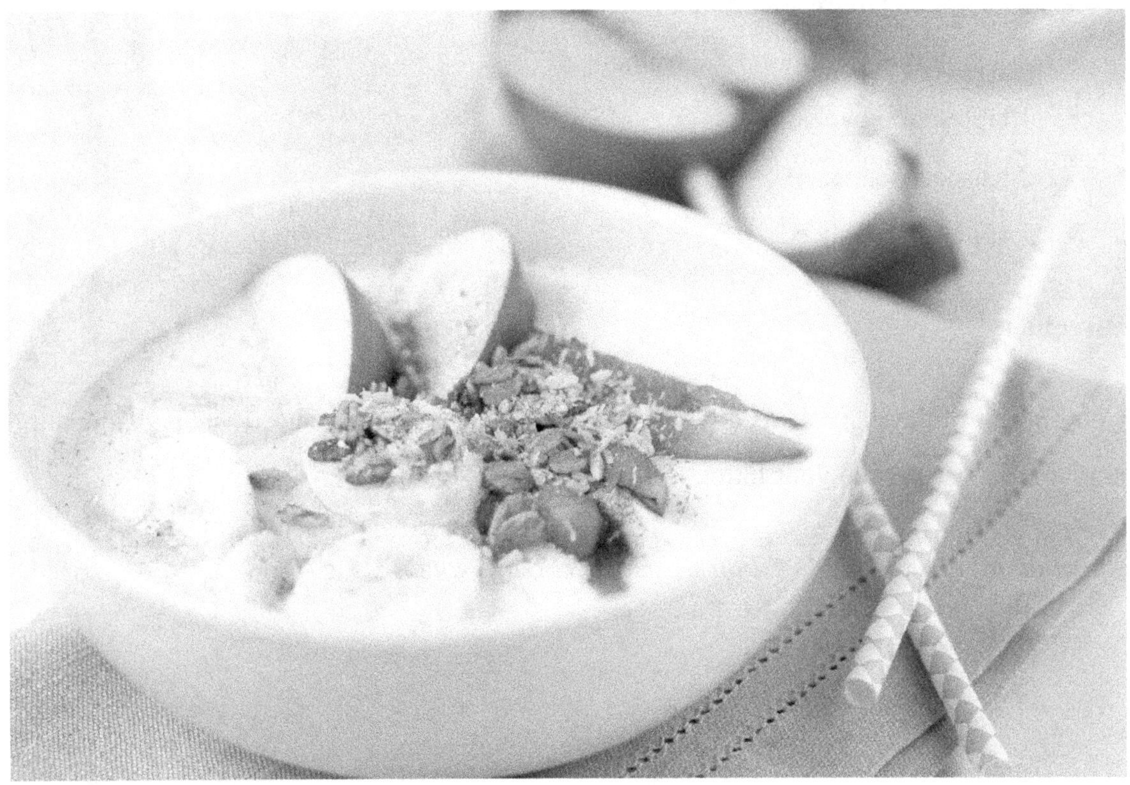

Prep Time: 5 minutes

Cooking Time: 2 minutes

Servings: 1 person

This recipe is very simple to prepare, just mix and it's ready. Packed with essential nutrients and vitamins, this recipe is a perfect dish for a super healthy breakfast during pregnancy.

Ingredients

- 1 cup plain Greek yogurt, unsweetened
- 2-3 tablespoons almonds or walnuts
- 1 tablespoon baobab
- 2 teaspoons stevia
- 1 apple, large, sliced

Directions

Combine all of the ingredients together in a large-sized mixing bowl. Taste and adjust the amount of sweetness to your likings

Nutritional Value: kcal: 464, Fat: 31 g, Fiber: 8 g, Protein: 11 g

Energy Breakfast

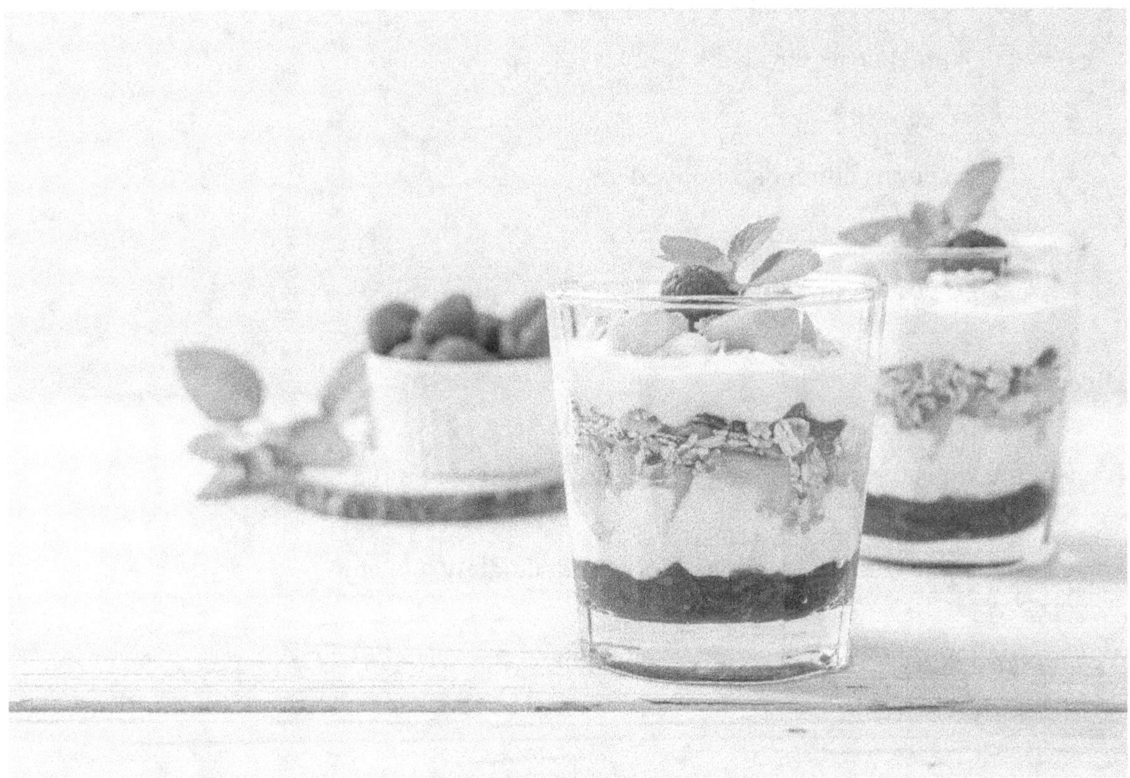

Prep Time: 2 minutes

Cooking Time: 2 minutes

Servings: 2 persons

If you are looking for a breakfast recipe with all the essential nutrients and max energy, then you must go for this one. You can even add raspberries to this recipe.

Ingredients

- 2 tablespoons dried apricots, chopped
- ¼ cup blueberries, fresh
- 1 cup cream of wheat
- 2 tablespoons almonds, chopped
- ¼ cup fresh strawberries, chopped
- 1 tablespoon brown sugar

Directions

Prepare the wheat cream per the instructions mentioned on the package.

Once done, top it with the toppings. Serve immediately and enjoy.

Nutritional Value: kcal: 410, Fat: 4.2 g, Fiber: 5.2 g, Protein: 11 g

Lunch & Dinner Recipes

Spinach Lamb Wraps

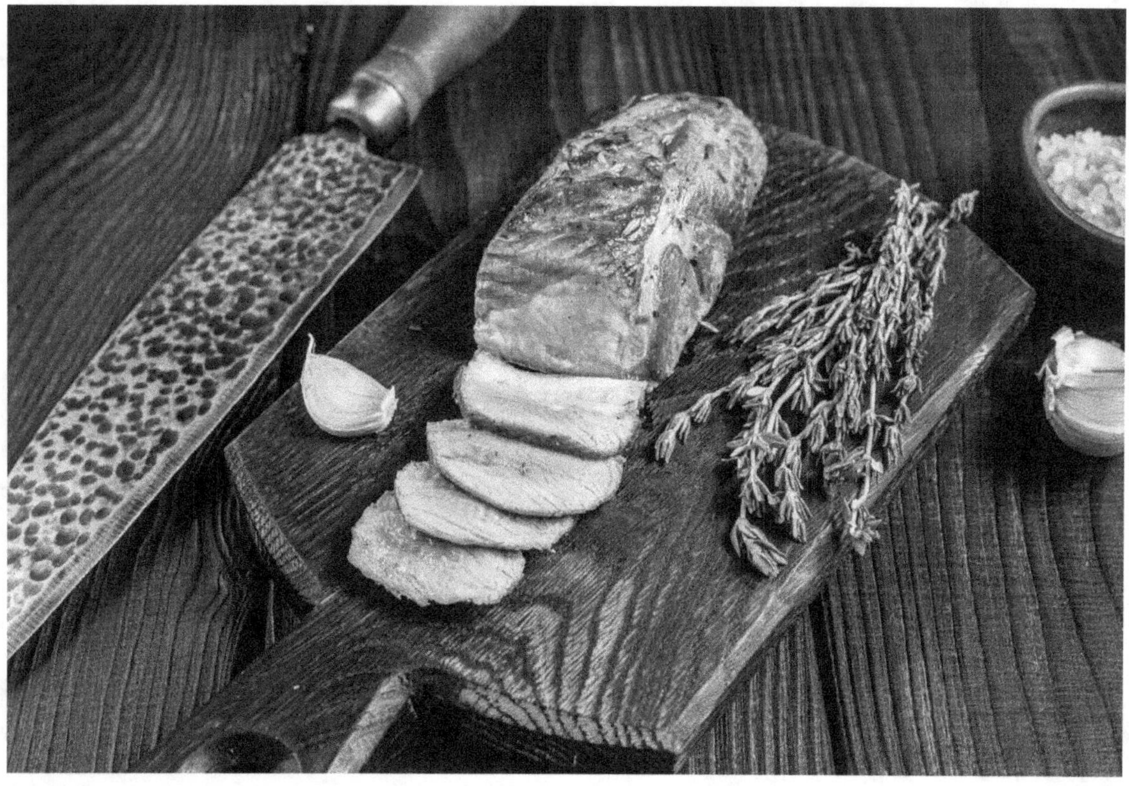

Prep Time: 20 minutes

Cooking Time: 20 minutes

Servings: 4 persons

One of the healthiest recipes that I have ever prepared for myself during the pregnancy period! You can serve the recipe as it is or with some chili ketchup on the side.

Ingredients

- 1 ¼ pounds lamb rump steaks, thinly sliced (fat trimmed)
- 4 spinach & herb wraps
- 1 packet taco seasoning (35g)
- 2 packets of beetroot with baby leaves salad mix (70g each)
- Olive oil, as required, to grease

Directions

Toss the meat with seasoning in a large-sized mixing bowl until nicely coated.

Next, coat a large, non-stick frying pan with olive oil and heat until hot, over medium heat. Work in batches and cook 1/3 of the coated lamb until tender, for a minute or two. Transfer to a large plate and repeat this cooking step with the leftover pieces of lamb.

Place a wrap on a clean work surface and then place ¼ of salad mix in the middle. Top with 1/3 of cooked lamb. Firmly roll up the wrap and ensure that the filling is enclosed. Repeat with the leftover lamb, salad mix and wraps to make four wraps in total. Once ready to serve, cut each wrap crossways into half.

Nutritional Value: kcal: 650, Fat: 31 g, Fiber: 3.2 g, Protein: 40 g

Tuna Pasta Bake

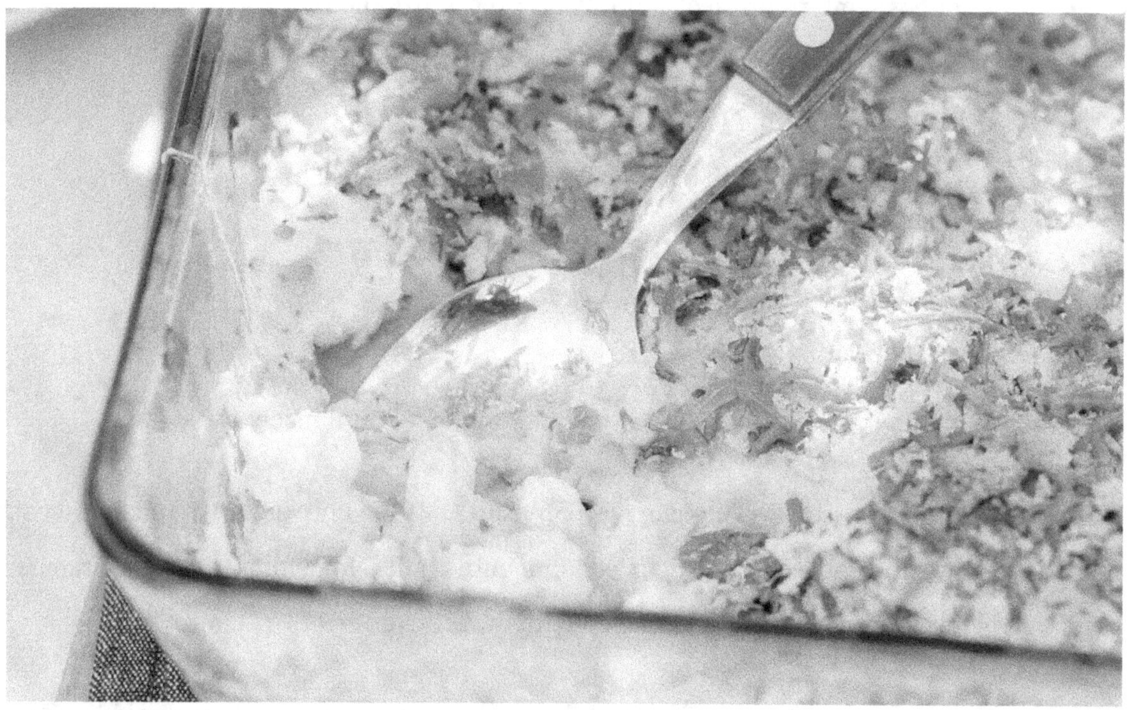

Prep Time: 10 minutes

Cooking Time: 30 minutes

Servings: 4 persons

I can guarantee you that you had never tasted this baked pasta before. It's quite easy to digest and tastes simply great. Just before baking, feel free to drizzle a bit of olive oil on the top.

Ingredients

- 1 can tuna (preferably in springwater), drained & flaked (approximately 1 pound)
- 2 cups milk, low-fat
- ¾ pounds macaroni pasta, dried
- 2 tablespoons plain flour
- 1 to 2 tablespoons softened butter
- ¾ cup low-fat pizza cheese, grated

Directions

Lightly coat an ovenproof dish (8 cup capacity) and then preheat your oven to 400 F in advance.

Next, prepare the pasta per the directions mentioned on the package until tender, in lightly salted boiling water. Drain, keep approximately ¼ cup of the cooking liquid aside and add pasta back to the pan.

Now, over medium heat in a large saucepan, heat up the butter until melted and then immediately add in the flour, cook until bubbling, for 1 minute, stirring frequently. Once done, remove the saucepan from heat and slowly stir in the milk until combined well. Place the saucepan back to the heat. Cook until the sauce boils & thickens, for 3 to 4 minutes, stirring every now and then. Remove from the heat and stir in ¼ cup of the cheese then, season with the pepper.

Add to pasta with reserved cooking liquid and tuna. Gently toss the ingredients until combined well. Fill the prepared dish with this mixture and then sprinkle with the leftover cheese. Bake in the preheated oven until the cheese is completely melted & turn golden, for 12 to 15 minutes. Serve immediately & enjoy.

Nutritional Value: kcal: 601, Fat: 16 g, Fiber: 2 g, Protein: 34 g

Banana Yoghurt Muffins

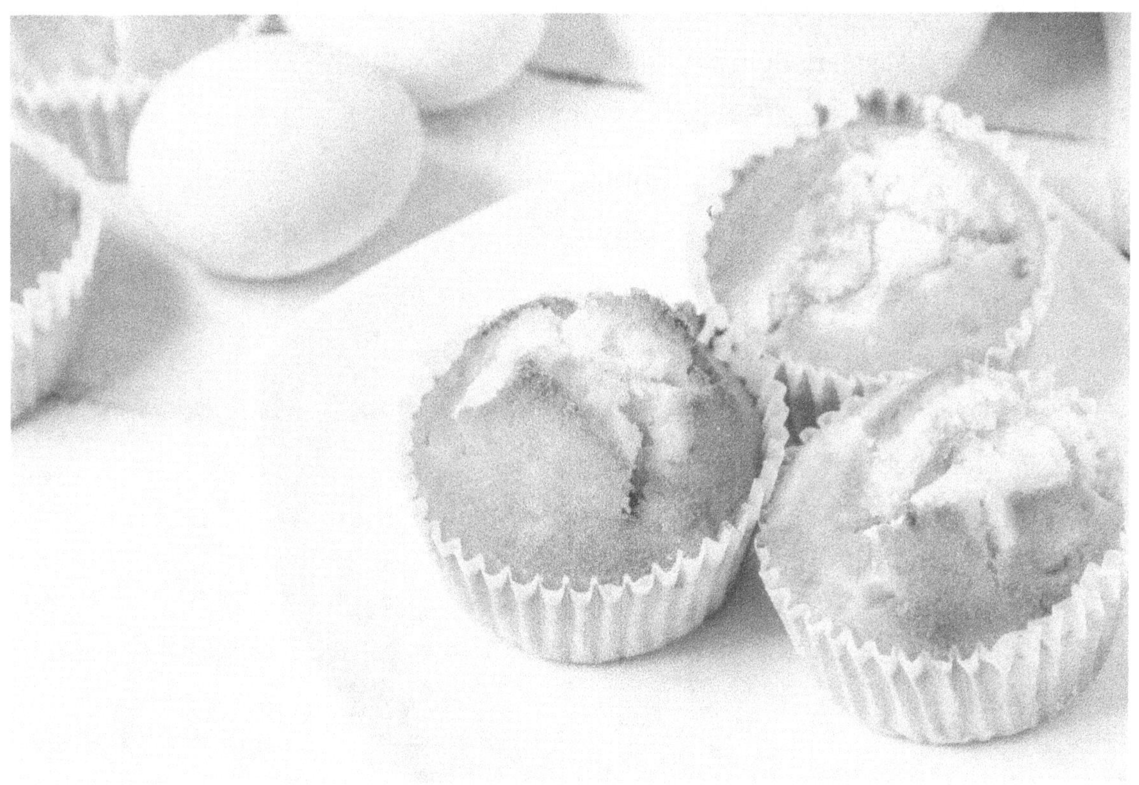

Prep Time: 20 minutes

Cooking Time: 30 minutes

Servings: 12 persons

Ingredients

- Absolutely delicious and easy to prepare! I served mine with a glass full of almond milk for added nutrition.
- Ingredients
- 1 ¾ cups flour, preferably self-rising
- 1 organic egg, large-sized
- ½ cup caster sugar
- 2 bananas, large & mashed
- 1 cup natural yoghurt
- 2/3 cup vegetable oil

Directions

Lightly coat a 12-hole, muffin pan (preferably with 1/3 cup capacity) and then preheat your oven to 350 F in advance.

Next, sift the flour with sugar in a large-sized mixing bowl until mixed well.

Combine the egg with yoghurt, 1 cup mashed banana and oil in a separate large-sized mixing bowl. Slowly add in the dry ingredients and continue to stir the ingredients until just combined.

Fill the coated muffin holes with the prepared mixture. Bake in the preheated oven until a skewer comes out clean, for 20 to 25 minutes.

Let the muffins to stand in a pan for a couple of minutes then transfer them to a wire rack to completely cool. Serve and enjoy.

Nutritional Value: kcal: 217, Fat: 11 g, Fiber: 1 g, Protein: 3.4 g

Ginger and Hoisin Chicken

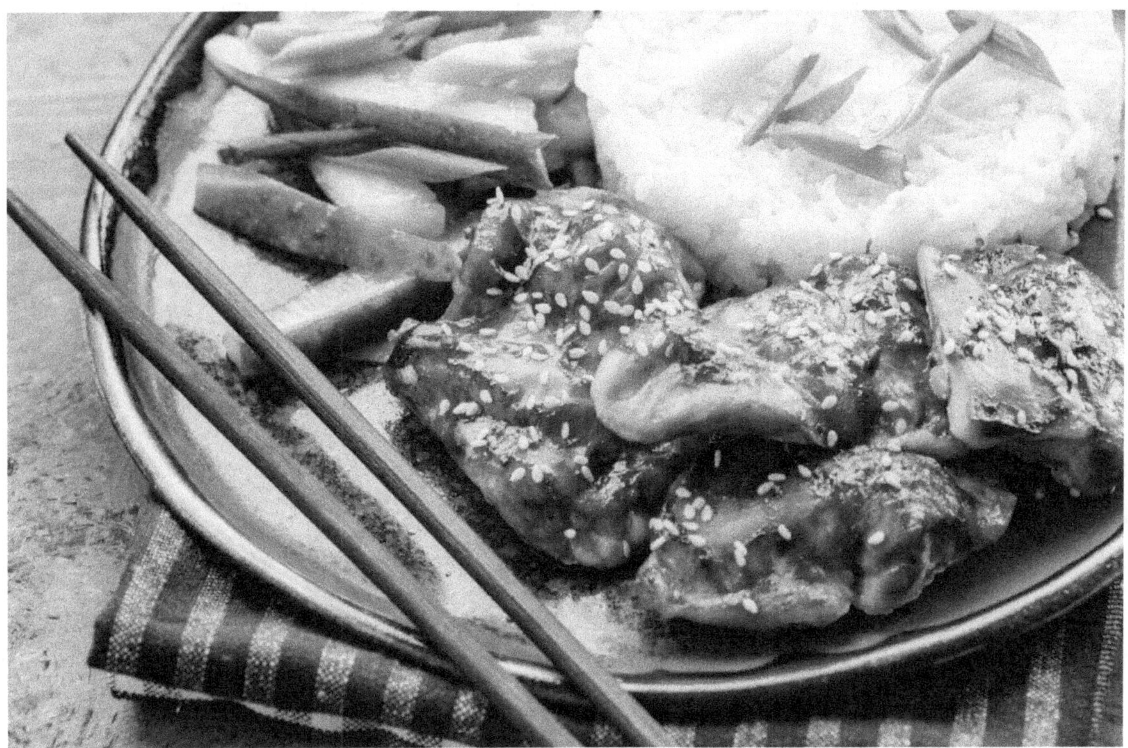

Prep Time: 10 minutes

Cooking Time: 30 minutes

Servings: 4 persons

Absolutely delicious and healthy! This recipe will keep you full for hours. Just before serving, you can sprinkle the dish with some sesame seeds.

Ingredients

- 1 ½ pounds chicken thigh fillets, trimmed olive oil cooking spray
- ¼ cup hoisin sauce
- 2 tablespoons soy sauce
- 1 tablespoon sesame seeds, toasted
- 2 teaspoons ginger, freshly-grated
- ½ pound snow peas, trimmed & sliced diagonally
- 4 green onions, sliced thinly
- ½ pound egg noodles, dried
- 2 tablespoons Chinese rice wine

Directions

Combine the soy sauce with hoisin sauce, ginger and rice wine in a jug. Next, add the chicken into a ceramic or shallow glass dish. Add half of the prepared sauce mixture. Once done, turn the chicken several times until nicely coated with the sauce. Cover & refrigerate for a couple of minutes.

Now, preheat your chargrill or barbecue plate (lightly coated with the oil) over high heat and then cook the coated chicken until browned & cooked through, for 3 to 4 minutes per side. Remove to a large plate. Cover & set aside for a couple of minutes then, slice it thinly.

In the meantime, prepare the noodles per the directions mentioned on the packet. During the last half a minute of your cooking time, add in the snow peas. Drain & remove to a large-sized serving bowl. Add the green onions & leftover sauce mixture. Give the ingredients a gently toss.

Top the noodle mixture with thinly sliced chicken. Just before serving, sprinkle the dish with some sesame seeds & enjoy.

Nutritional Value: kcal: 328, Fat: 16 g, Fiber: 4 g, Protein: 32 g

Honey, Ginger & Lemon Pork Stir-Fry

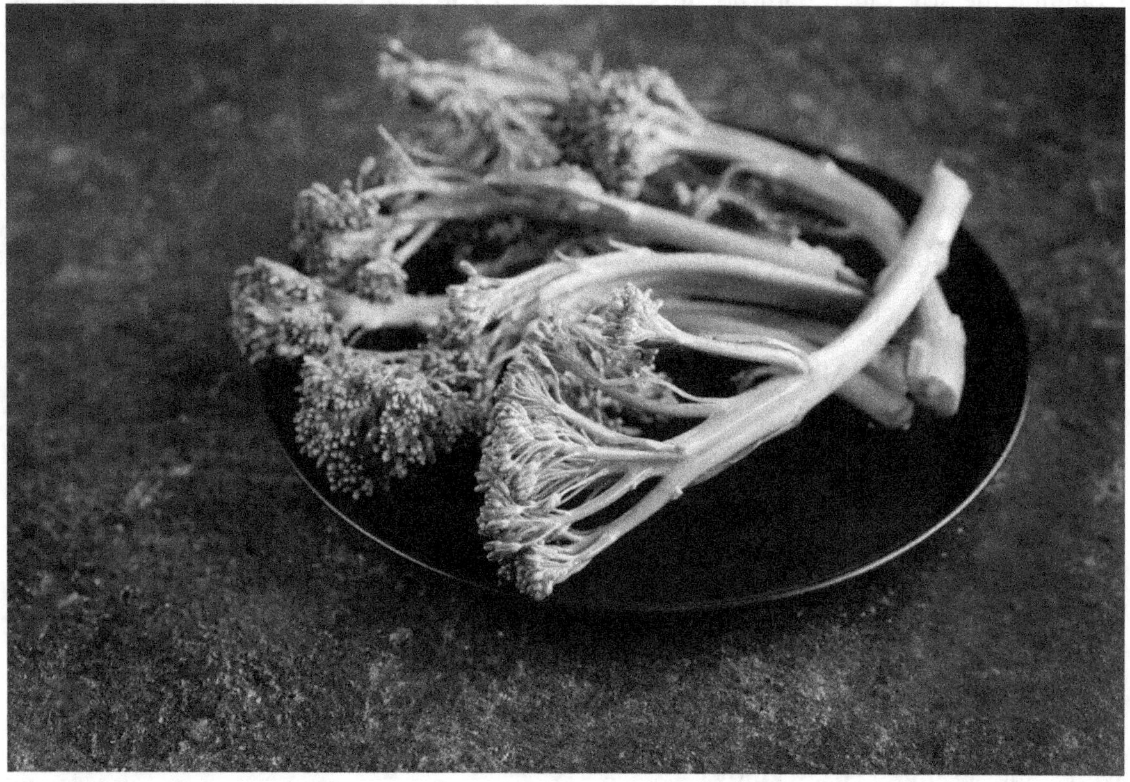

Prep Time: 20 minutes

Cooking Time: 20 minutes

Servings: 4 persons

This is one of my favorite snack recipes and full of flavors. I sure that you will love it too. Feel free to top your dish with freshly squeezed lime juice.

Ingredients

- 2 bunches broccolini, trimmed, halved
- 1 ¼ pounds pork stir-fry strips
- 2 tablespoons soy sauce
- 1 garlic clove, crushed
- 3 teaspoons corn flour
- 2 tablespoons honey
- Juice of 1 lemon, freshly squeezed
- 2 tablespoons Chinese rice wine
- 3cm piece ginger, grated finely
- 2 tablespoons vegetable oil
- Steamed white rice, to serve

Directions

Combine the meat with ginger and garlic in a large-sized mixing bowl until mixed well.

Next, over high heat in a wok, heat up half of the oil until hot, swirl to coat the bottom completely. Once done, add half of the pork & stir-fry until browned, for 2 to 3 minutes and then remove to a large-sized mixing bowl. Repeat with the leftover pork and oil.

Combine honey with lemon juice, rice wine and soy sauce in a jug. Place corn flour into a small-sized mixing bowl and then slowly add in the sauce mixture, give the ingredients a good stir until completely smooth.

Add the pork back to the wok and then add in the Broccolini, stir-fry the ingredients for a minute or two and then stir in the corn flour mixture. Bring the mixture to a boil & continue to stir-fry the ingredients until sauce thickens and the broccolini and pork both are just cooked through, for 2 to 3 more minutes. Serve hot with the rice and enjoy.

Nutritional Value: kcal: 448, Fat: 16 g, Fiber: 8.8 g, Protein: 24 g

Strawberry and Spinach Salad

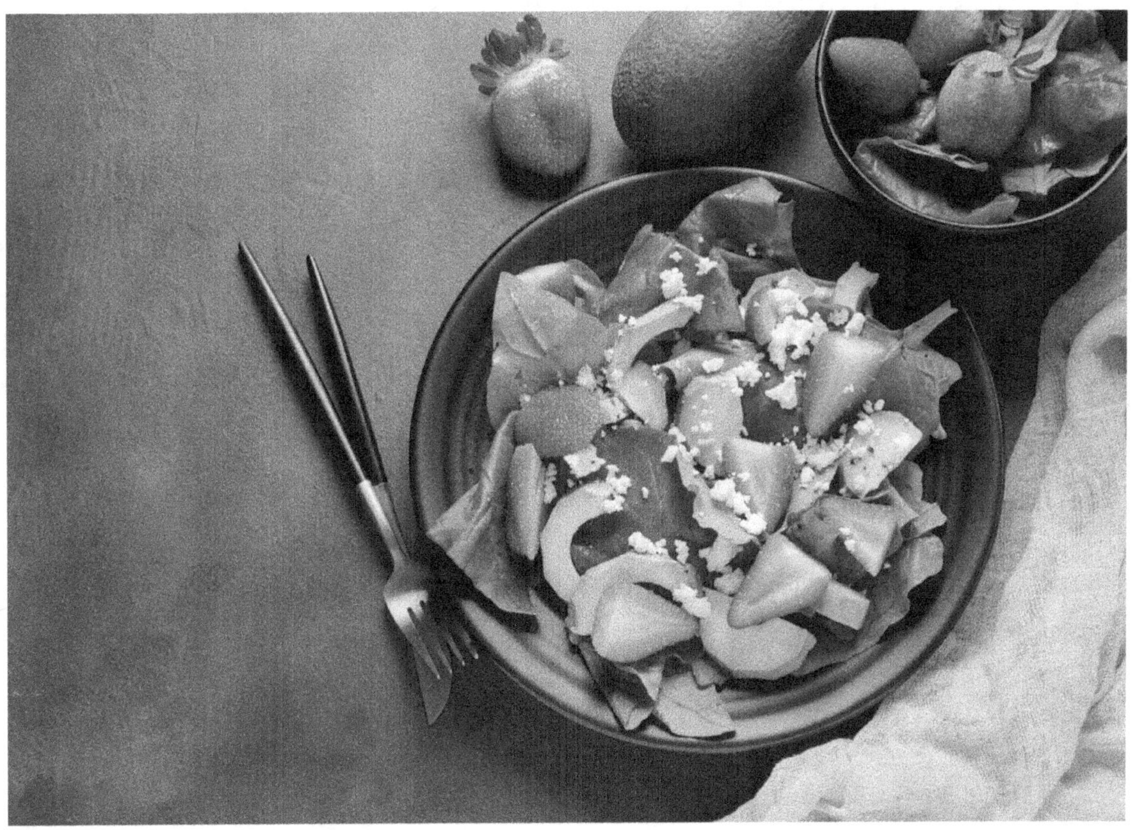

Prep Time: 10 minutes

Cooking Time: 10 minutes

Servings: 4 persons

This healthy fresh salad recipe is a perfect dish for summers. For a tangy flavor, feel free to squeeze some fresh lemon on the top and enjoy.

Ingredients

- 150g soft Goats' Cheese
- 1 pound fresh strawberries
- 130g Walnuts
- ½ pound fresh spinach leaves
- Juice of 1 lime, fresh
- 2 to 3 tablespoons olive oil plus more for frying
- 1 teaspoon dried parsley
- Black pepper and salt, to taste

Directions

Over moderate heat in a wok or large frying pan, heat up a bit of oil until hot. Once done, add & sauté the walnuts for a minute or two, until burnt slightly, let cool and then chop it roughly.

Wash & hull the fresh strawberries then slice.

Next, rip the spinach leaves gently and then add the leaves with strawberries and walnuts into a large-sized mixing bowl.

Gently mash the goat's cheese with hands and sprinkle on top of the salad.

For Dressing: Whisk lime juice with olive oil and parsley and then season with a bit of pepper and salt. Once done, pour this mixture on top of the salad, toss the ingredients gently, serve immediately and enjoy.

Nutritional Value: kcal: 434, Fat: 34 g, Fiber: 4.6 g, Protein: 12 g

Salmon & Spinach Quinoa Salad

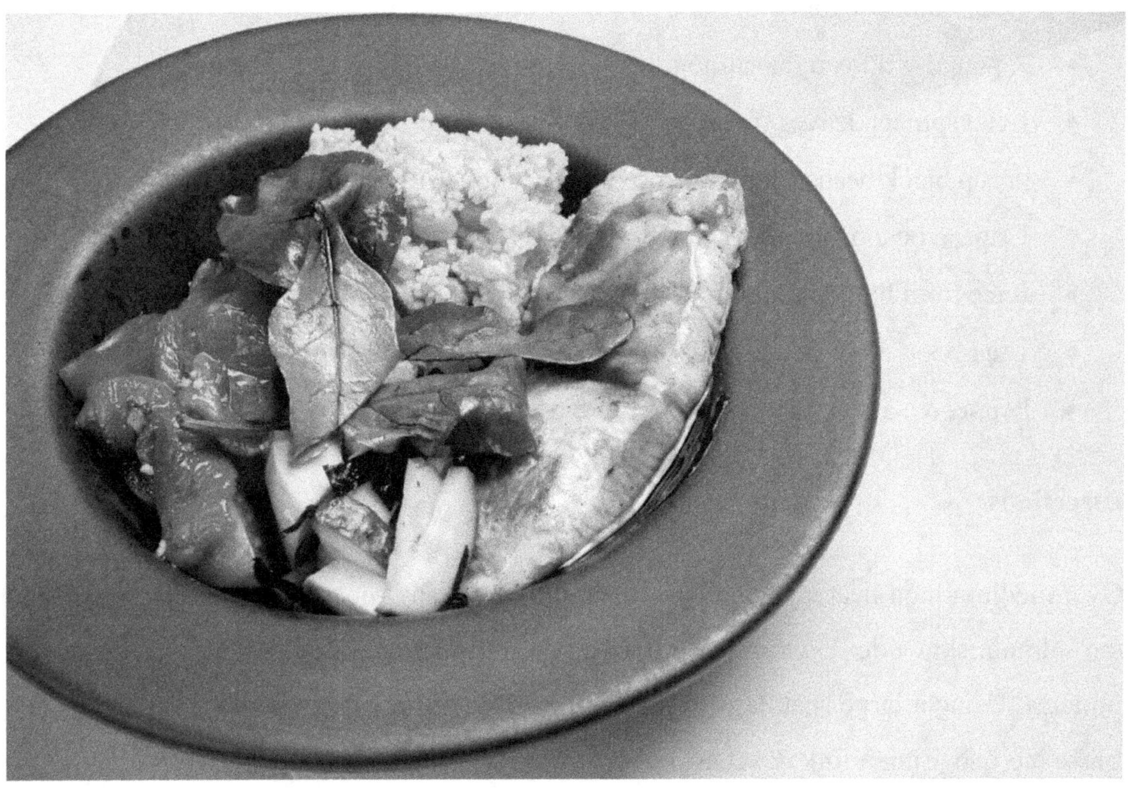

Prep Time: 10 minutes

Cooking Time: 10 minutes

Servings: 2 persons

This recipe is super hearty and tastes awesome. The combination of quinoa and salmon makes this recipe a hit. A nice way to get protein with added nutrients!

Ingredients

- 1 cup quinoa, cooked
- ½ pound wild-caught salmon
- 1 cup spinach leaves, fresh
- ½ cup black beans (drain & rinsed well), cooked
- 1 ripe avocado, sliced
- Juice from half a lemon, fresh
- 1 teaspoon olive oil
- Pepper & salt, to taste

Directions

Over medium-high heat in a small pan, heat up the oil until hot. Once done, carefully add the salmon, skin side down into the hot pan & cook until turn golden brown, for 3 to 4 minutes. Using a large spatula, flip the salmon & cook the other side for 2 to 3 minutes. Flake the fish using a fork & set aside.

Next, add the black beans, quinoa, spinach leaves and avocado slices to a large-sized mixing bowl and then top with the salmon pieces. Once done, add in the fresh lemon juice & mix well. Season with pepper and salt, to taste. Serve immediately and enjoy.

Nutritional Value: kcal: 568, Fat: 30 g, Fiber: 11 g, Protein: 29 g

Ultimate Pregnancy Burger

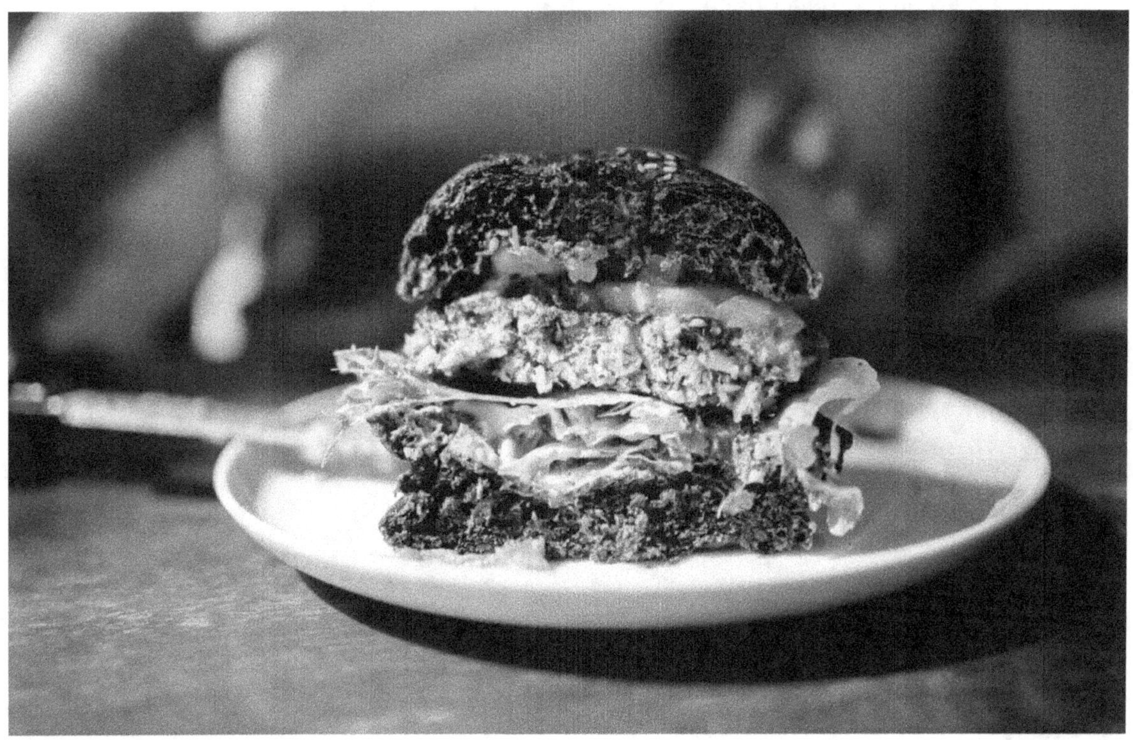

Prep Time: 20 minutes

Cooking Time: 20 minutes

Servings: 5 persons

The best part about this recipe is that it's gluten-free and plant-based. For added nutrients, feel free to add avocado slices to it.

Ingredients

- 1 cup green lentils, cooked
- ½ cup sweet onion, diced
- 1 cup carrots, grated
- 5 oz mushrooms, roughly chopped
- 1 cup rolled oats
- 1 tablespoon ground flaxseeds
- 2 handfuls fresh spinach (approximately 2 cups)
- 1 tablespoon olive oil, divided
- 1 teaspoon each of paprika, garlic powder, dried parsley, and salt

For Serving:

- sliced red onion
- sliced tomato
- sliced avocado
- gluten-free burger bun
- vegan mayo drizzle

Directions

Cook the lentils per the instructions mentioned on the package.

Next, grate the carrots in a food processor using the disc attachment, set aside until ready to use.

Now, over moderate heat in a large cast-iron pan, heat up a teaspoon of olive oil until hot. Once done, add & cook the chopped onion until translucent, for a couple of minutes, stirring frequently. Then immediately, add in the grated carrots and chopped mushrooms. Combine parsley with garlic powder, paprika, and salt. Give the ingredients a good stir & continue to cook for 5 minutes with lid on.

Next, blend the rolled oats and ground flaxseeds in the food processor until the flour consistency is achieved, reserve approximately 2 tablespoons of oat / flaxseed mixture, set aside until ready to use.

Add vegetables, spinach, and lentils from the pan into the food processor, pulse until mixed well and you get sticky mixture.

Next, heat up a bit of oil more into the same pan. Make five burgers from the prepared mixture, sprinkling the bottom and top with the kept-aside oat / flaxseed flour. Carefully cook the formed burgers until each side turn golden brown, with the lid on, flipping, as required. Form your burgers with the buns & toppings of your choice. Serve immediately & enjoy.

Nutritional Value: kcal: 160, Fat: 12 g, Fiber: 4.1 g, Protein: 8 g

Delicious Mouth-watering Frittata

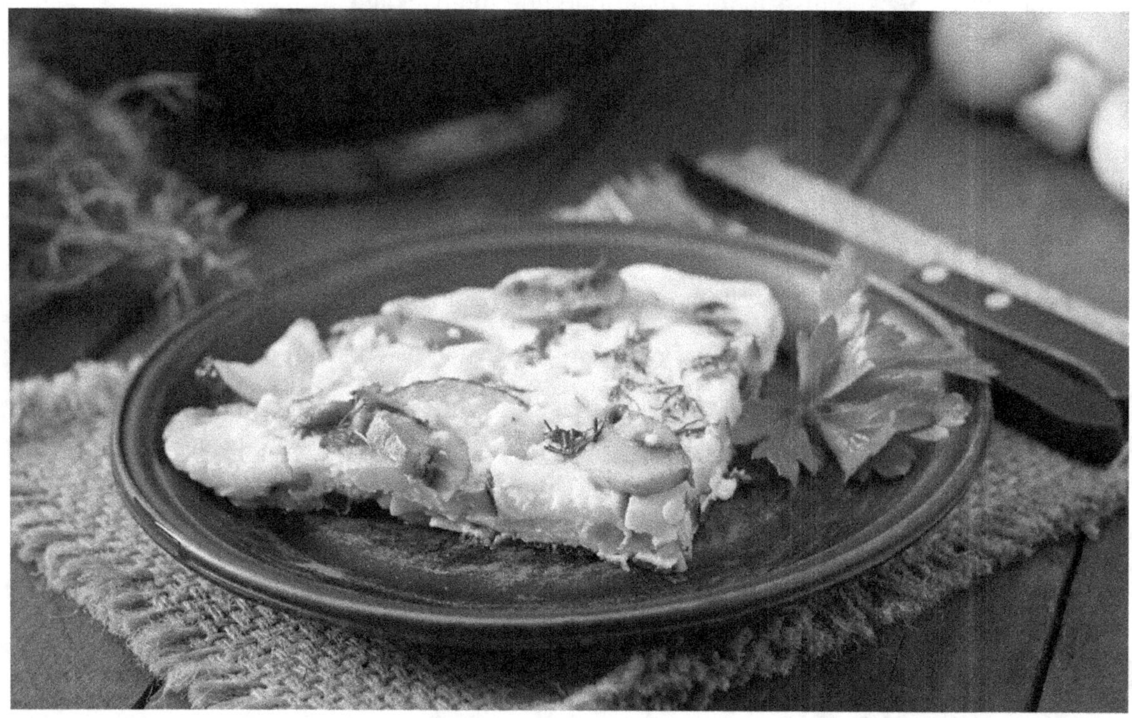

Prep Time: 10 minutes

Cooking Time: 30 minutes

Servings: 8 persons

This recipe is packed with healthy nutrients and tastes delicious too. You can serve this recipe as a breakfast, lunch, or even dinner. You can use any of your favorite unsweetened milk in this recipe. Feel free to garnish your recipe with sliced green onion.

Ingredients

- 12 organic eggs, large-sized
- ½ cup almond milk, unsweetened
- ¼ cup green onion tops, diced
- 1 teaspoon smoked paprika
- 2 small zucchini, diced
- 1 bell pepper, diced
- ¼ teaspoon black pepper
- 2 tablespoons extra virgin olive oil
- 1 teaspoon sea salt

Directions

Preheat your oven to 350 F in advance.

Next, over medium heat in a medium to large-sized oven safe skillet, heat up the olive oil until hot. Add the zucchini and bell pepper. Sautee the ingredients for 3 to 5 minutes, until soft.

Add the green onion, black pepper, smoked paprika and salt.

Next, whisk the eggs with the almond milk in a large-sized mixing bowl. Pour the prepared egg mixture with vegetables into the hot pan, cook until the sides are just firm, for 3 to 5 minutes.

Place the pan in the preheated oven & bake until everything is set, for 20 more minutes.

Serve hot and enjoy.

Nutritional Value: kcal: 140, Fat: 10 g, Fiber: 0.7 g, Protein: 8 g

Banana Bread

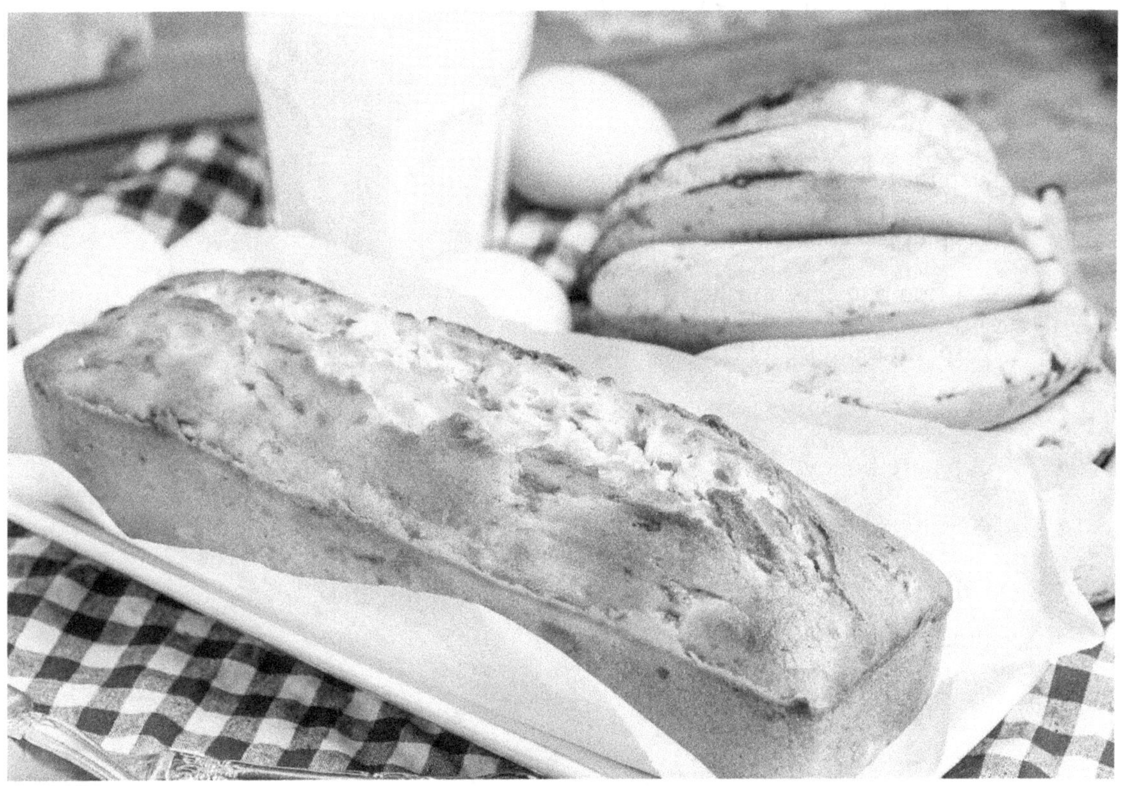

Prep Time: 20 minutes

Cooking Time: 40 minutes

Servings: 1 large loaf

This recipe tastes great when served warm. This gluten-free bread has only got natural sugars and no oils or fat. Feel free to add a few chocolate chips to this recipe to make this bread sweeter.

Ingredients

- 1 ½ cups rice flour (gluten-free) plus ½ teaspoon xanthum gum
- ½ cup gluten-free rolled oats
- 2 ½ teaspoons baking powder
- 1 heaping teaspoon of ground cinnamon
- 1/3 cup apple sauce
- 3 to 4 ripe bananas, mashed
- 1 teaspoon baking soda
- 2 organic eggs, large
- ½ cup pure honey
- 2 teaspoons vanilla extract
- ¼ cup coconut oil
- A pinch of sea salt

Directions

Preheat your oven to 350 F in advance

Next, combine all of the dry ingredients together in a large-sized mixing bowl until mixed well.

Combine the leftover ingredients in a separate bowl until combined well.

Mix the mixture of wet into the mixture of dry ingredients until blended well.

Coat a 9" Pyrex with the coconut oil & lightly dust with the flour

Fill the prepared pan with the batter, evenly distributing using a large spatula

Place in the center rack of your preheated oven & bake until a toothpick comes out clean, for 30 to 40 minute.

Nutritional Value: kcal: 188, Fat: 7 g, Fiber: 3 g, Protein: 19 g

Sweet Potato and Lentil Soup

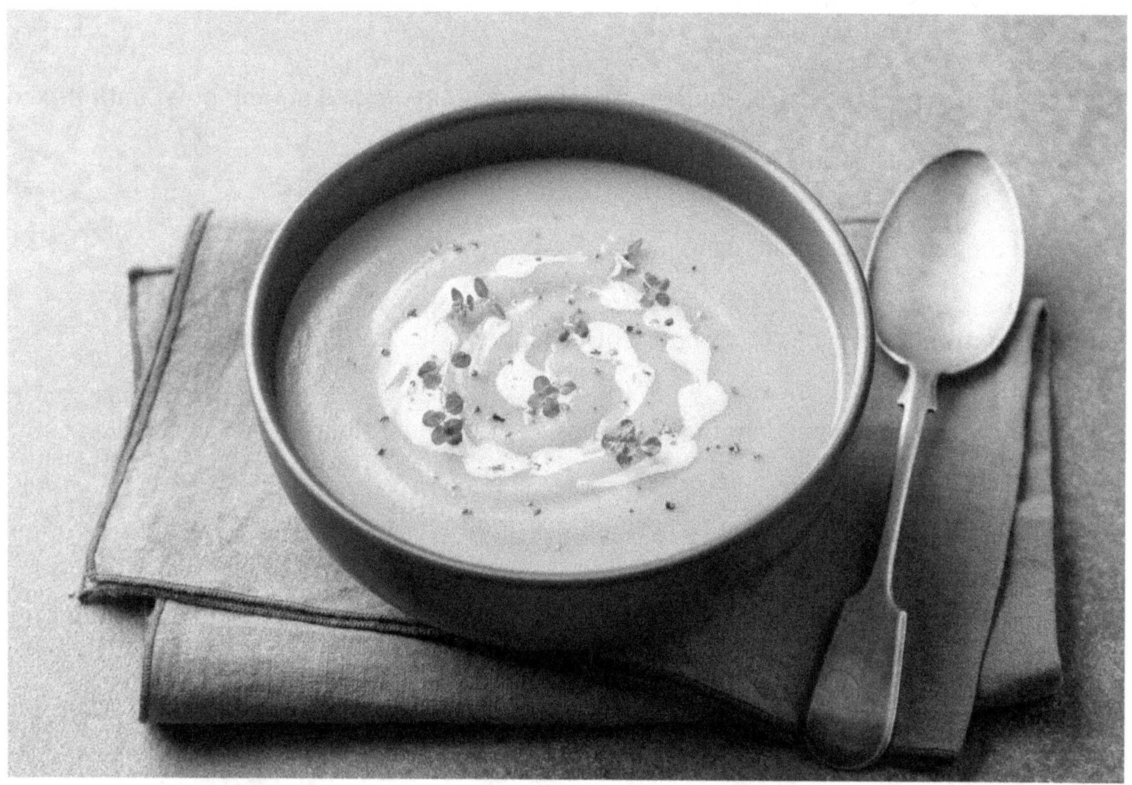

Prep Time: 10 minutes

Cooking Time: 30 minutes

Servings: 6 persons

Absolutely delicious and healthy! I served mine with some bread buns.

Ingredients

- 2 pounds sweet potato
- 1 eating apple, peeled, cored & grated
- 2 onions, grated
- 20g pack of coriander, stalks chopped
- 2 Liters vegetable stock
- 2 teaspoons curry powder
- 3 garlic cloves, crushed
- 300ml milk
- ¼ pound red lentils
- juice of 1 lime, fresh
- 3 tablespoons olive oil
- Fresh root ginger (thumb-sized piece), grated

Directions

Toast the curry powder over moderate heat in a large saucepan for a minute or two and then add in the olive oil, stirring frequently.

Tip in the ginger, onions, garlic, apple, and coriander stalks then, gently season and cook for 5 minutes, stirring frequently.

In the meantime, peel & grate the sweet potatoes. Once done, immediately tip it into the hot pan with milk, lentils, stock and seasoning, cover and bring it to a simmer, continue to cook for approximately 20 minutes.

Once done, blend the soup carefully using a stick blender until smooth. Stir in the freshly squeezed lime juice, taste and adjust the amount of seasoning, if required. Serve immediately, top with fresh coriander leaves (roughly chopped).

Nutritional Value: kcal: 196, Fat: 16 g, Fiber: 2 g, Protein: 1.2 g

Chicken and Broccoli

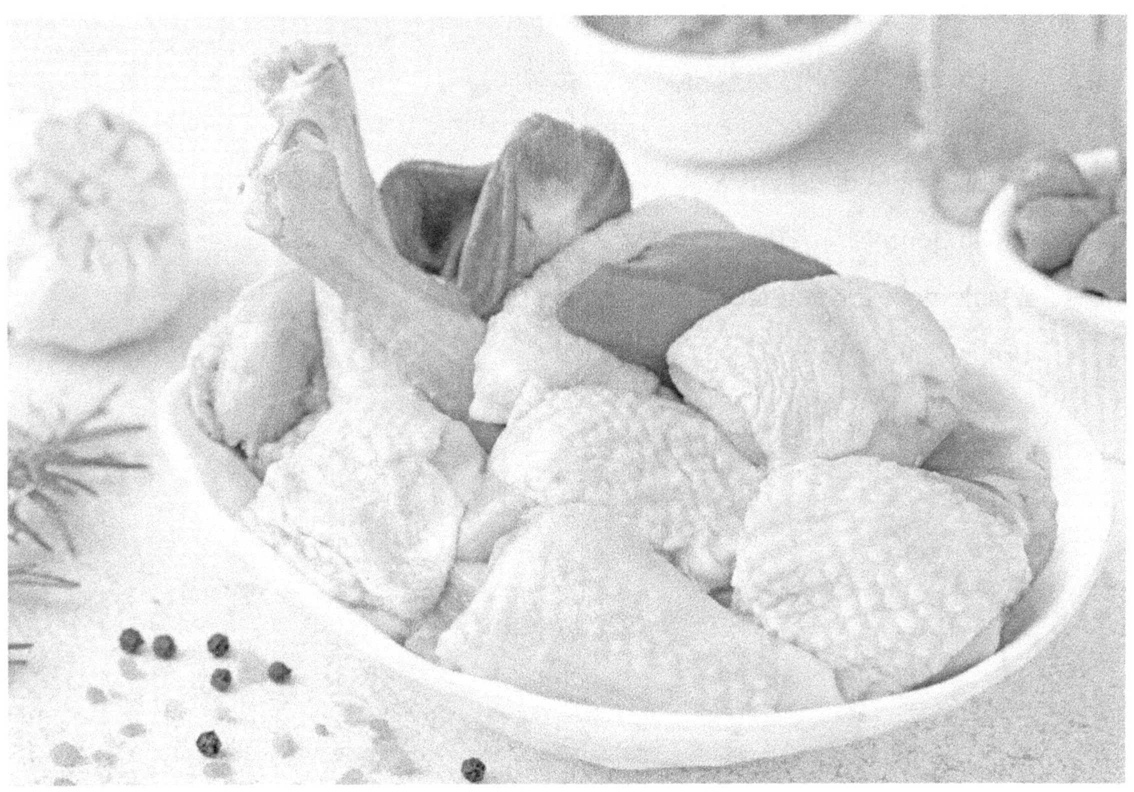

Prep Time: 20 minutes

Cooking Time: 40 minutes

Servings: 4 persons

My whole family loves this recipe a lot. Just before serving, top this dish with freshly chopped lemongrass and then sprinkle with a pinch of ground black pepper. Serve hot and enjoy.

Ingredients

- 3 oz. butter
- 1½ pounds fresh broccoli
- 3 ½ pounds chicken
- 2 tablespoons dry sherry
- ⅓ cup flour
- 2 tablespoons parmesan cheese, grated plus more
- Boiling salted water
- ½ cup single cream
- Pepper & salt, to taste

Directions

Steam the chicken for a couple of minutes, until tender, drain well and reserve approximately 2 cups of the cooking liquid. Remove the bones from chicken and then cut the meat into small-sized pieces, keep hot.

Discard any large part of the stalks from fresh broccoli & most of the leaves. Put in the boiling salted water & cook for 12 to 15 minutes, drain & keep hot.

Next, over moderate heat in a large pan, heat up the butter until melted and then stir in the flour, cook for a minute. Remove from the heat & slowly add in the reserved liquid, mix the ingredients until blended well. Return to the heat & bring it to a boil, continue to cook the ingredients until the sauce boils & thickens, stirring frequently.

Stir in the sherry and cream, season with pepper and salt to taste. Arrange the broccoli at the bottom of your ovenproof dish, pour approximately half of the prepared sauce on top. Arrange the chicken pieces on top of the sauce.

Add parmesan cheese to the leftover sauce and then pour over the chicken. Sprinkle with a bit of more parmesan cheese. Place under the griller (broiler) until sauce starts to bubble and is lightly browned. Serve immediately and enjoy.

Nutritional Value: kcal: 170, Fat: 6.2 g, Fiber: 6.0 g, Protein: 3.2 g

Quinoa Paneer Patties

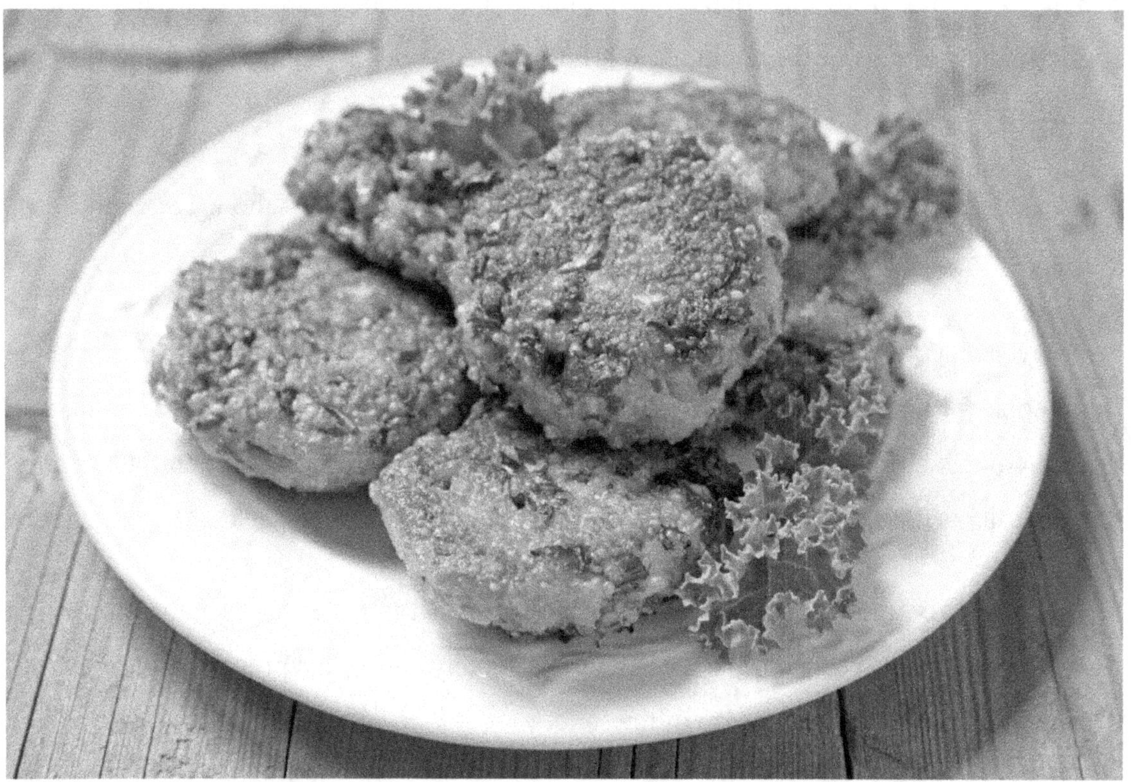

Prep Time: 10 minutes

Cooking Time: 30 minutes

Servings: 10 persons

These healthy cutlets are very high in protein. Just serve these patties with freshly prepared mint chutney, chopped cucumber, and carrot and enjoy the taste.

Ingredients

- 1 cup Paneer, grated

- Ghee/ oil for brushing

For Pressure Cooking:

- 1 raw banana, washed, pricked & cut into half
- ½ cup pre-washed quinoa, uncooked
- 1 cup water
- A pinch of salt

For Green Masala:

- A fistful of fresh mint leaves
- ½ cup peanuts without skin, roasted
- 1 " knob of ginger or ½ tablespoon grated
- 2 green chilis or adjust to your spice level
- A fistful of cilantro leaves / coriander
- Other Spices
- 1 teaspoon cumin powder
- 2 teaspoon fresh lemon juice
- A few twists of black pepper
- ½ teaspoon garam masala, optional
- Salt to taste

For the Dip

- ½ " piece of ginger
- 1 green chili
- ½ cup mint, packed
- 2 to 3 tablespoons yogurt
- ½ cup cilantro, packed
- Salt to taste

Directions

Add a cup of water to the inner pot and then place the trivet on it.

Next, place quinoa, 1 cup water & salt in the safe bowl of your Instant Pot.

Cover with lid & place the sliced potato on top of it.

Secure the lid to its place and switch on the Instant Pot.

Pressure cook manually for 3 minutes on high pressure.

Once done, wait for 10 minutes and let the pressure to release naturally then perform a quick release feature.

Carefully the lid, remove the quinoa and potato slices, let completely cool.

In the meantime grate the paneer, prepare the green masala and dip.

For Green Masala

Blend the coriander with mint, green chilies and roasted skinned peanuts.

Grate the paneer using a fine grater attachment in a food processor, preferably for 8 to 10 seconds.

Let the cooked potato and quinoa to completely cool down before proceeding with the recipe.

For a lump free mixture, peel & grate the potato.

Putting it together

Combine all of the ingredients together and then add in the spices.

Next, over moderate heat in a large skillet, heat up the oil or ghee until hot.

Make approximately ¼" thick and 2" broad patties from the prepared mixture.

Carefully place the formed patties into the hot skillet. Decrease the heat to low and cook the patties until crispy & golden brown, for 2 to 3 minutes, flipping gently mid-way.

Serve warm with a freshly chopped salad & dip on side. Enjoy.

For Green Chutney:

Blend all of the ingredients together in a blender until completely smooth.

Taste & adjust the amount of seasoning, if required.

Nutritional Value: kcal: 165, Fat: 2.5 g, Fiber: 12 g, Protein: 14 g

Conclusion

Thank you again for reading this book.

You don't need to worry about the nutritional level since you would be getting enough of it with all the recipes in this e-book.

As mentioned earlier, avoid eating papaya, pineapple, and grapes throughout your pregnancy period.

It's important for you to consult your doctor often about the overall growth of your little one and for added vitamins/minerals as well.

What are you still waiting for? If you haven't bought this book till now then, do it now and forget about the nutritional level for your little one.

About the Author

Born in New Germantown, Pennsylvania, Stephanie Sharp received a Masters degree from Penn State in English Literature. Driven by her passion to create culinary masterpieces, she applied and was accepted to The International Culinary School of the Art Institute where she excelled in French cuisine. She has married her cooking skills with an aptitude for business by opening her own small cooking school where she teaches students of all ages.

Stephanie's talents extend to being an author as well and she has written over 400 e-books on the art of cooking and baking that include her most popular recipes.

Sharp has been fortunate enough to raise a family near her hometown in Pennsylvania where she, her husband and children live in a beautiful rustic house on an extensive piece of land. Her other passion is taking care of the furry members of her family which include 3 cats, 2 dogs and a potbelly pig named Wilbur.

Watch for more amazing books by Stephanie Sharp coming out in the next few months.

Author's Afterthoughts

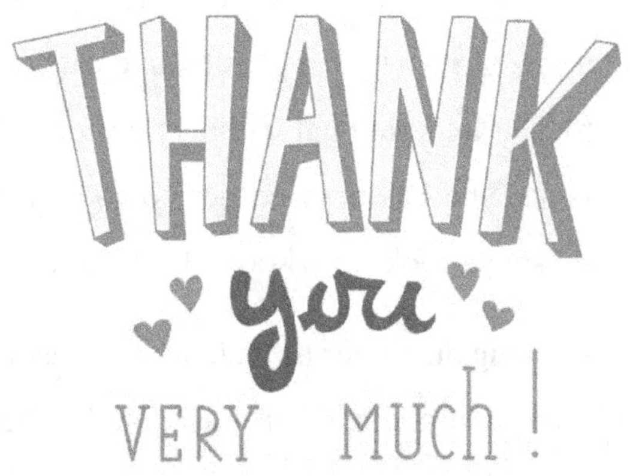

I am truly grateful to you for taking the time to read my book. I cherish all of my readers! Thanks ever so much to each of my cherished readers for investing the time to read this book!

With so many options available to you, your choice to buy my book is an honour, so my heartfelt thanks at reading it from beginning to end!

I value your feedback, so please take a moment to submit an honest and open review on Amazon so I can get valuable insight into my readers' opinions and others can benefit from your experience.

Thank you for taking the time to review!

Stephanie Sharp

For announcements about new releases, please follow my author page on Amazon.com!

You can find that at:

https://www.amazon.com/author/stephanie-sharp

*or Scan **QR-code** below.*